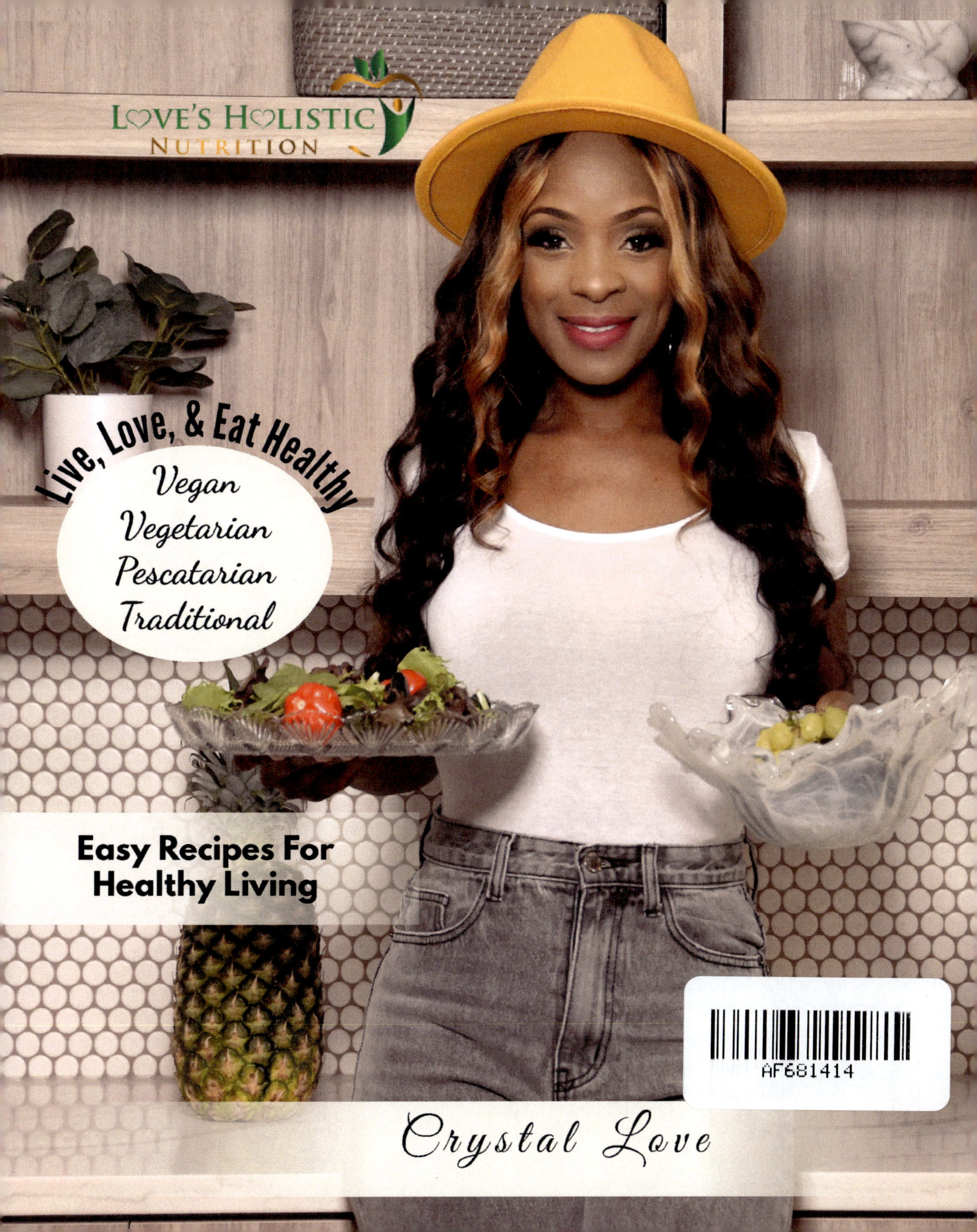
LOVE'S HOLISTIC
NUTRITION
Live, Love, & Eat Healthy
Vegan
Vegetarian
Pescatarian
Traditional
Easy Recipes For
Healthy Living
Crystal Love

ISBN: 978-1-955297-01-1

Library of Congress Control Number: 2021920736

Title Your Truth Publishing
9103 Woodmore Centre #334
Lanham, MD 20706
www.titleyourtruthpublishing.com

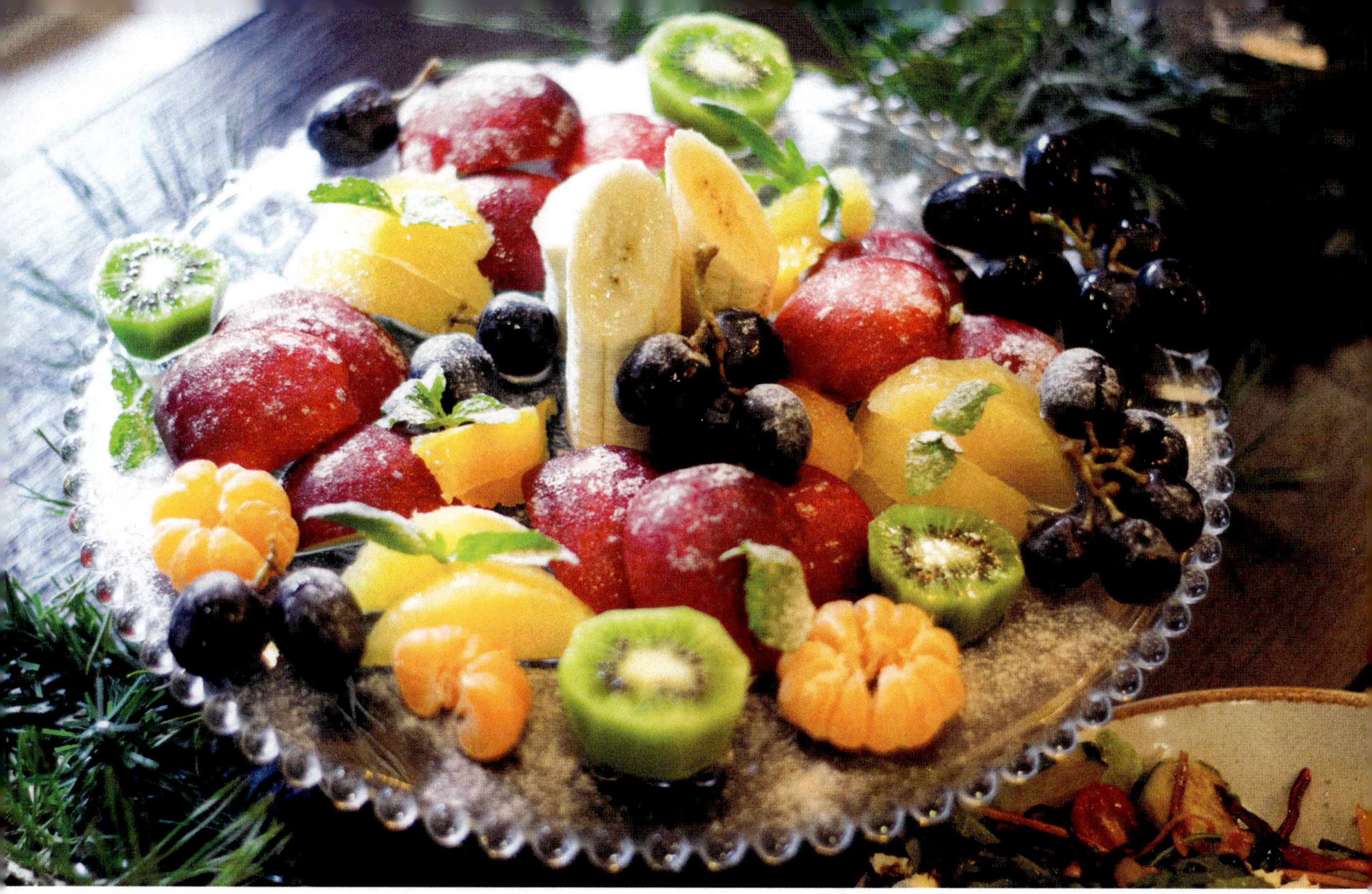

*Welcome to your new healthy lifestyle!*

Healthy eating is vital to your overall well-being and effectiveness in every area of your life. How you are feeling physically, mentally, emotionally, and socially can sometimes be affected by your diet. I began my journey to healthy eating over 20 years ago, and it has been a rewarding one. I realized that healthy eating is a lifestyle. Sometimes, when you develop eating habits based upon a specific goal, it can often lead to cycles of disappointment when that goal doesn't meet your expectations. This is only the beginning, as you begin your healthy eating regimen by choosing a diet plan that suits you. A special bonus has been included for you in the back of the book. There, you will find a daily food journal, as well as a creative space for you to discover your own recipes. Have fun on this new healthy eating journey!

LOVE'S HOLISTIC NUTRITION

# CONTENTS



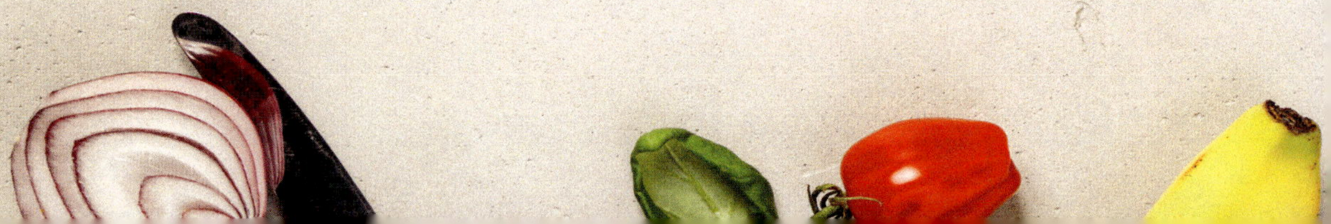

# CONTENTS

# *Breakfast Recipes*

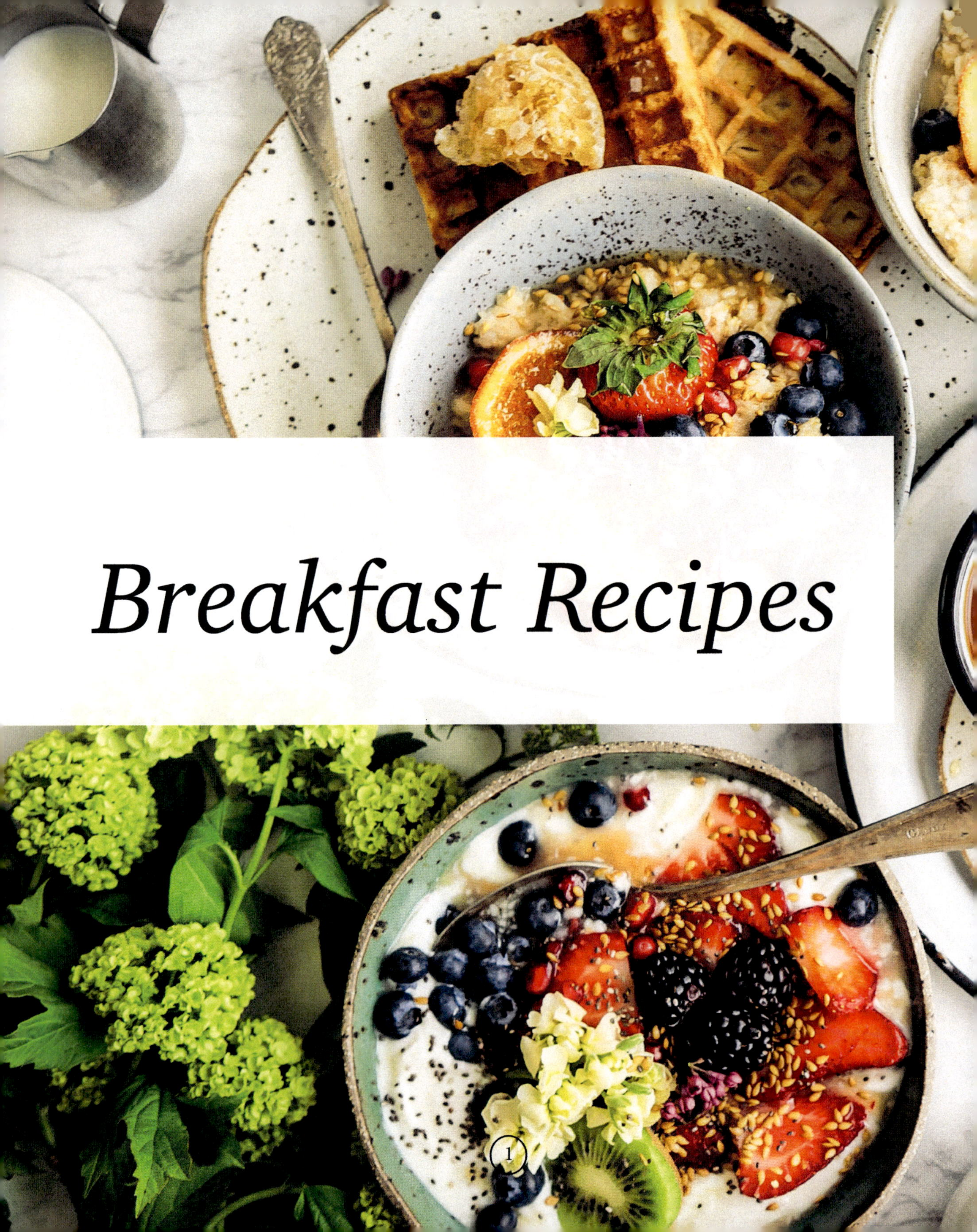

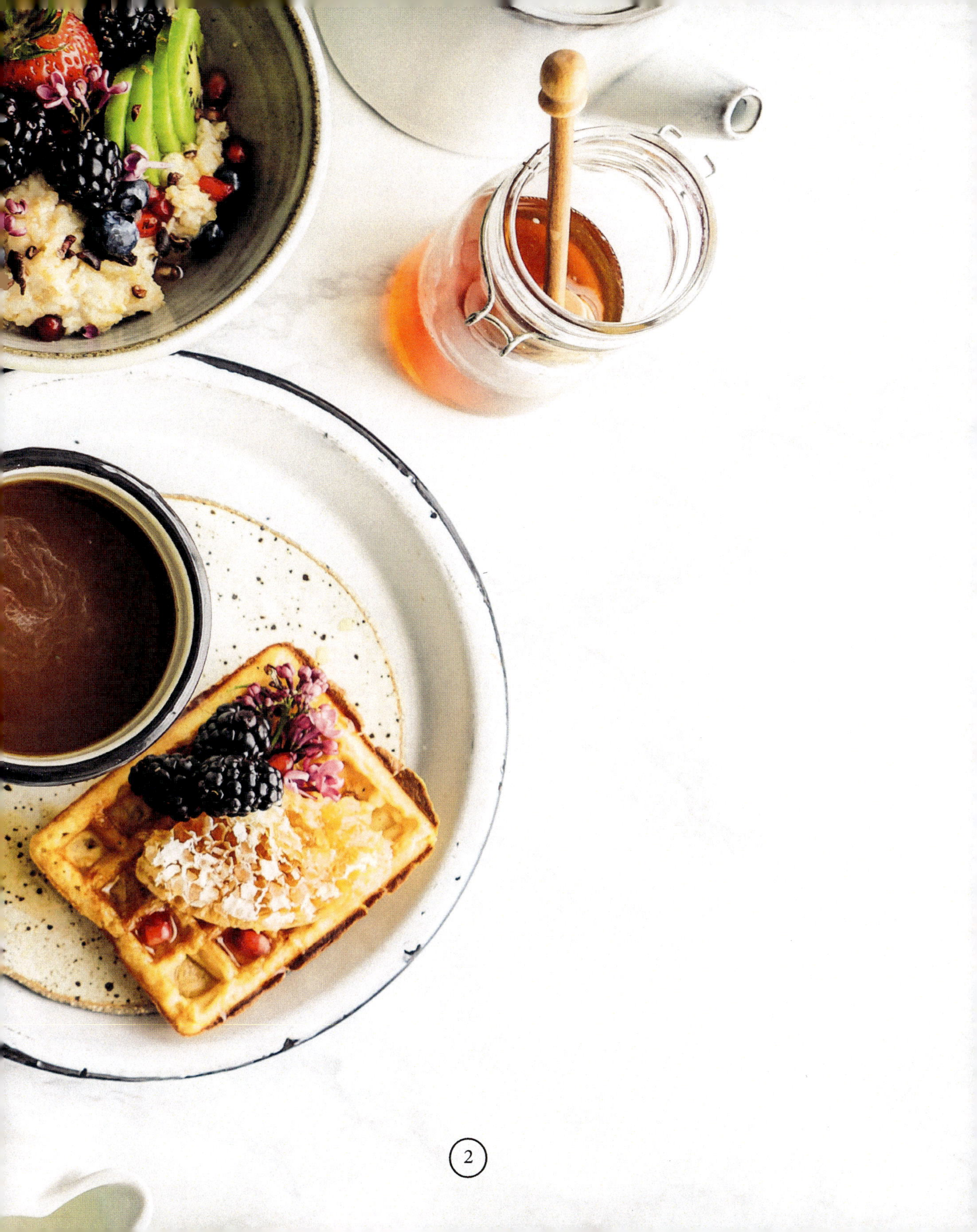

# Apple Carrot Muffin

**Nutritional Info**

*Calories: 257 kcal | Carbohydrates: 51.6 g | Protein: 3.1 g | Fat: 4.9 g*
*Total Preparation Time: 4 minutes | Serves: 12*

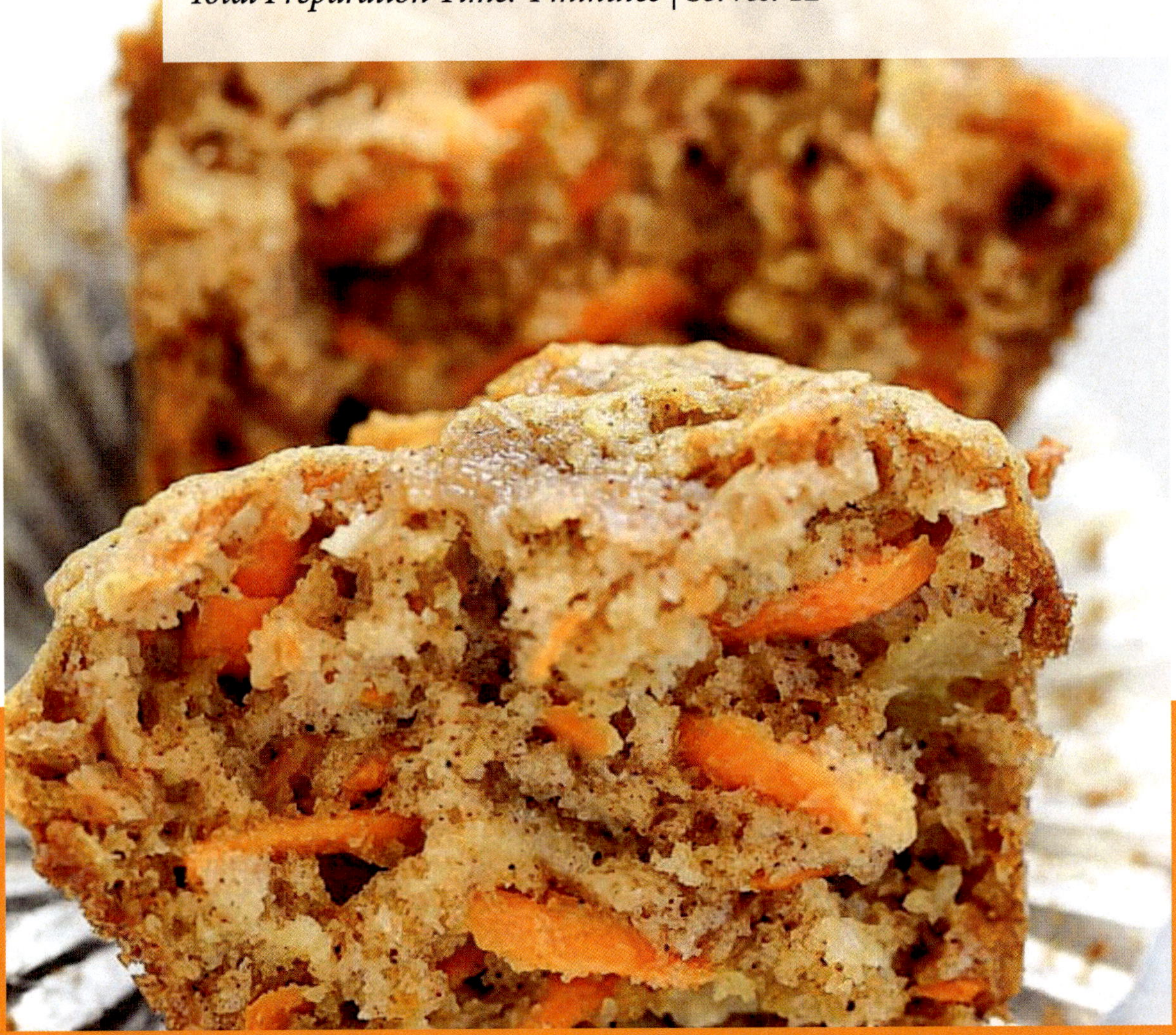

# INGREDIENTS

- *4 tsp. of baking soda*
- *1 tsp. of baking powder*
- *1 cup of brown sugar*
- *4 tsp. of ground cinnamon*
- *2 tsp. of salt*
- *2 cups of finely grated carrots*
- *½ cup of white sugar*
- *2 large apples- peeled, cored, and shredded*
- *2 tbsp. of egg replacer (dry)*
- *1¼ cups of applesauce*
- *4 tbsp. of vegetable oil*
- *2 ½ cups of all-purpose flour*

# DIRECTIONS

1. Preheat oven to 375°F (190°C).
2. Line the muffin cups with paper liners.
3. Combine the brown sugar, white sugar, flour, baking soda, baking powder, cinnamon, and salt in a large mixing basin.
4. Combine the carrots and apples in a large mixing bowl.
5. Whisk together the egg substitute, applesauce, and oil in a small bowl.
6. Combine the wet and dry components.
7. Drop the batter into prepared pans.
8. Bake for 20 minutes in a preheated oven.
9. Allow 5 minutes for muffins to cool in pans before removing to cool completely.
10. Serve and enjoy!

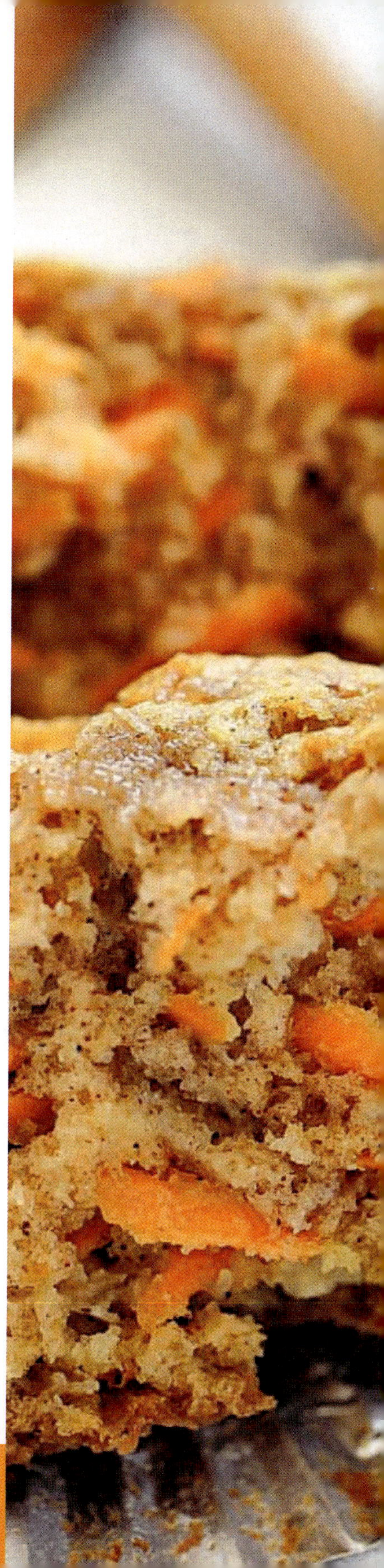

# *Mango Craze Juice Blend*

***Nutritional Info:***

*Calories: 15 kcal | Carbohydrates: 38.4 g | Protein: 1.3 g | Fat: 0.6 g*
*Total Preparation Time: 1 minute | Serves: 4*

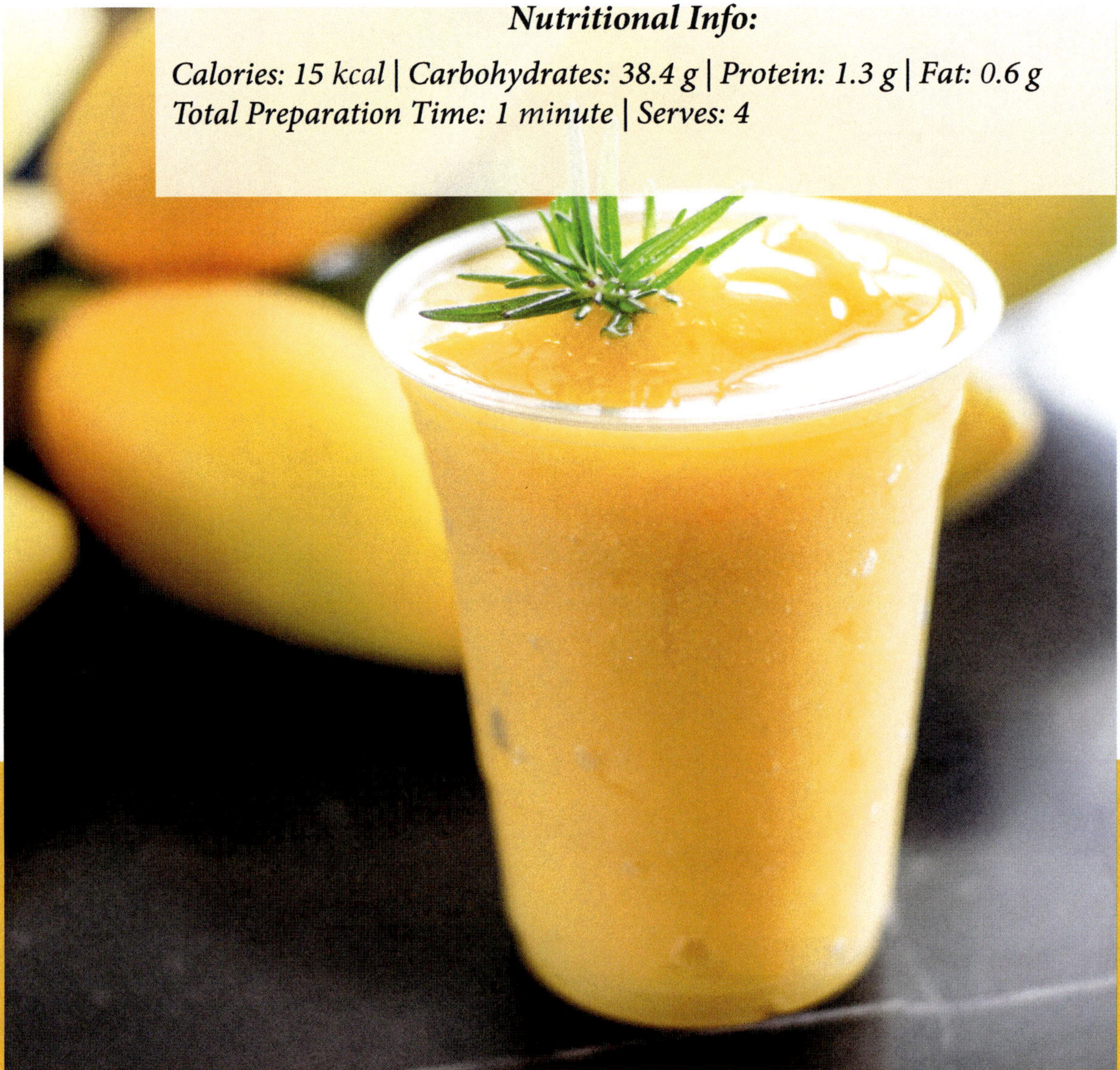

# *INGREDIENTS*

- *3 cups of mango chunks*
- *1½ cups of fresh or frozen peach slices*
- *¼ cup of orange segments, chopped*
- *¼ cup of nectarines, pitted and diced*
- *½ cup of orange juice*
- *1 cup of ice cubes*

# *DIRECTIONS*

1. Mix all of the ingredients in a high-power blender.
2. Blend on the "high" setting for 3-4 minutes.
3. Add more orange juice if the mixture looks too thick.
4. Pour the drink mixture into 4 serving glasses.
5. Serve and enjoy!

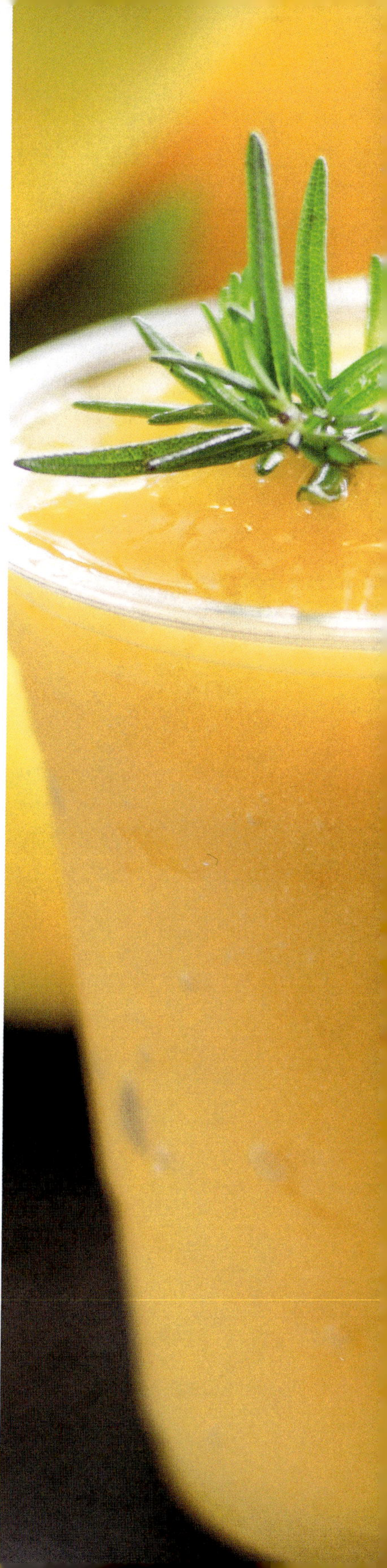

# Nectarine Sunshine Smoothie

**Nutritional Info:**

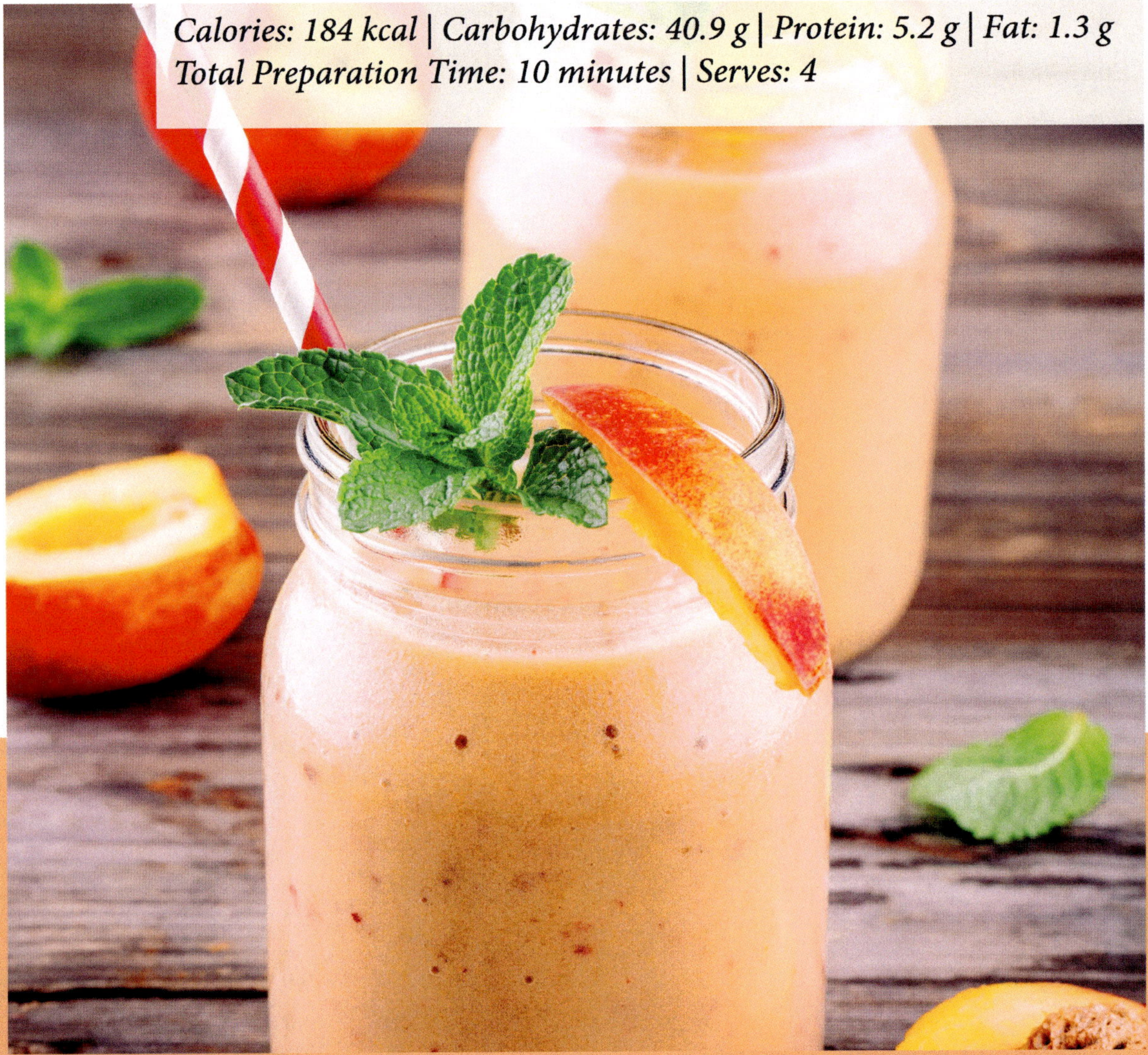

*Calories: 184 kcal | Carbohydrates: 40.9 g | Protein: 5.2 g | Fat: 1.3 g*
*Total Preparation Time: 10 minutes | Serves: 4*

# *INGREDIENTS*

- *1 cup of vanilla coconut yogurt*
- *4 small nectarines, pitted and quartered*
- *2 small oranges, peeled and quartered*
- *1 cup of fresh orange juice*
- *1 tbsp. of honey*
- *1 frozen banana, sliced*

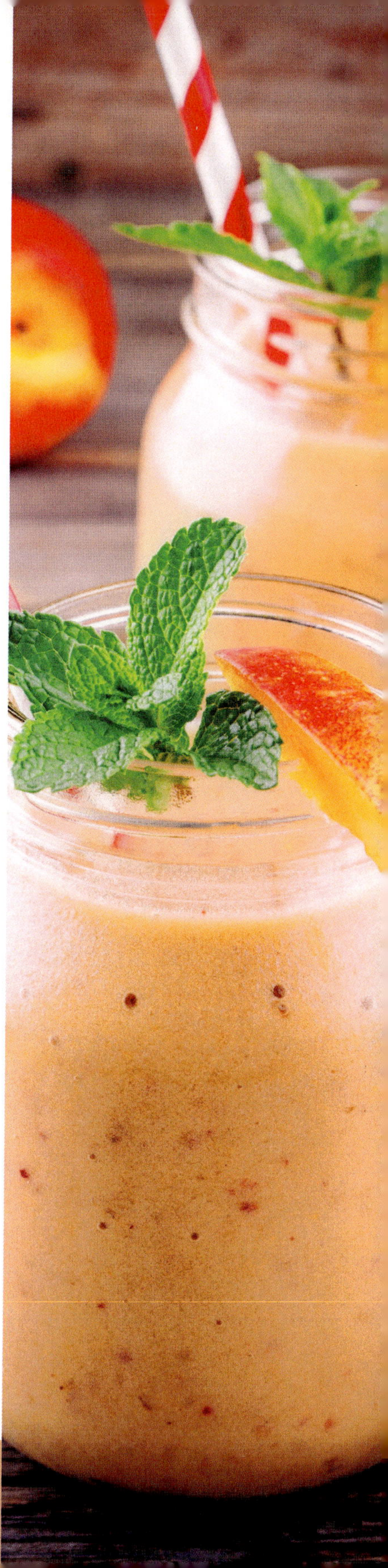

# *DIRECTIONS*

1. Mix all of the ingredients in a high-power blender.
2. Blend on the "high" setting for 3-4 minutes.
3. Add more orange juice if the mixture looks too thick.
4. Strain the drink mixture into 4 serving glasses.
5. Serve and enjoy!

# *Vegan Steel Cut Oats with Apples and Cinnamon*

***Nutritional Info:***

*Calories: 110 kcal | Carbohydrates: 19.4 g | Protein: 2.7 g | Fat: 2.9 g*
*Total Preparation Time: 35 minutes | Serves: 6*

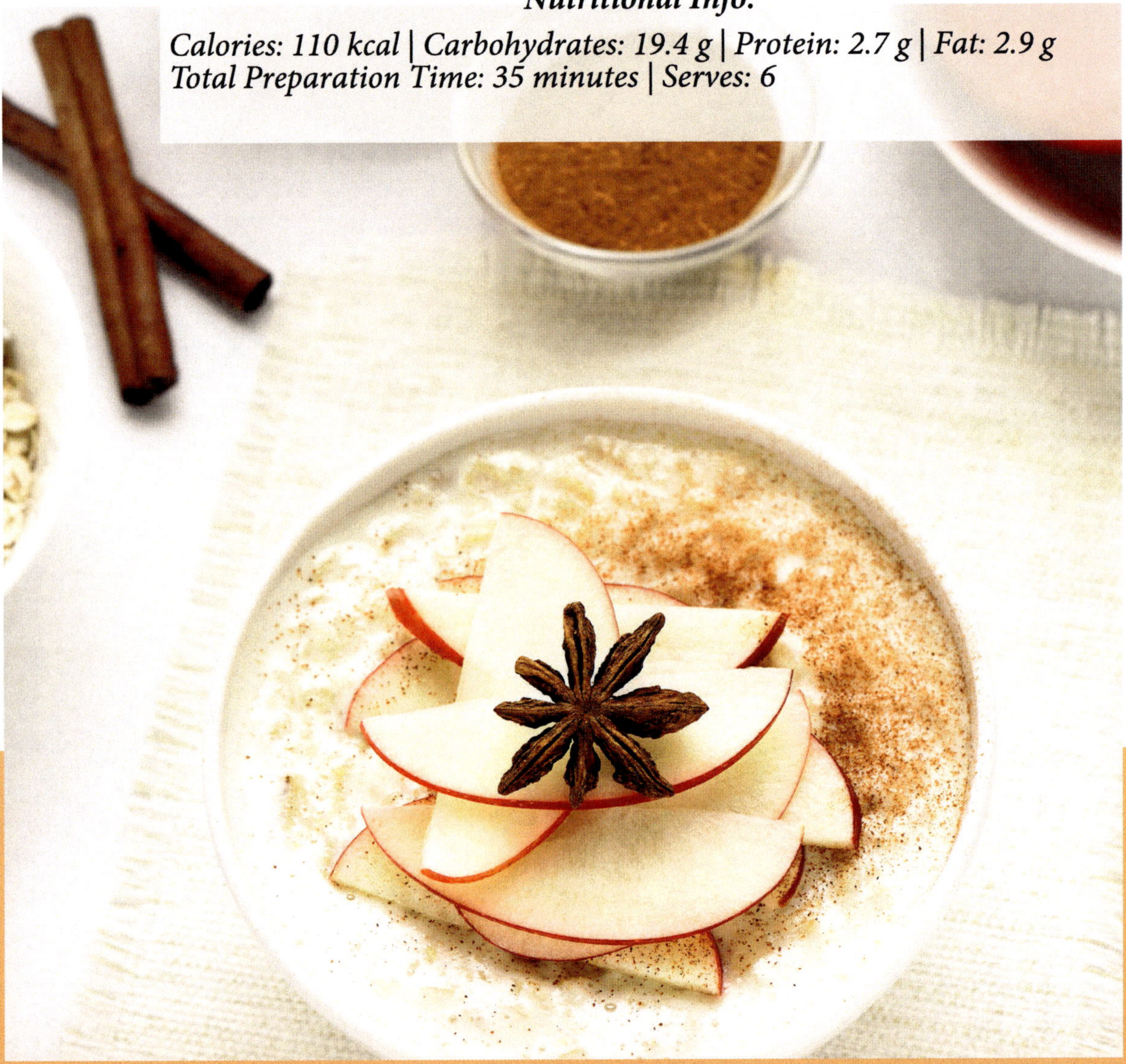

# *INGREDIENTS*

- *2 tbsp. of maple syrup*
- *2 tbsp. of flaxseed meal*
- *1 apple, chopped*
- *1 cup of almond milk*
- *1 tsp. of ground cinnamon*
- *1 cup of steel cut oats*
- *1 tbsp. of almonds, chopped*
- *2 cups of water*

# *DIRECTIONS*

1. In a multi-functional pressure cooker, combine the water, almond milk, oats, maple syrup, flaxseed meal, apple, cinnamon, and almonds.
2. Secure the lid by closing and locking it.
3. Select the high pressure, as directed by the manufacturer.
4. Set the timer for a minimum of 10 minutes to allow time for the pressure to build.
5. After the pressure builds, release it naturally, using the manufacturer's instructions.
6. Remove the lid by unlocking it.
7. Thoroughly mix the oatmeal.
8. Serve and enjoy!

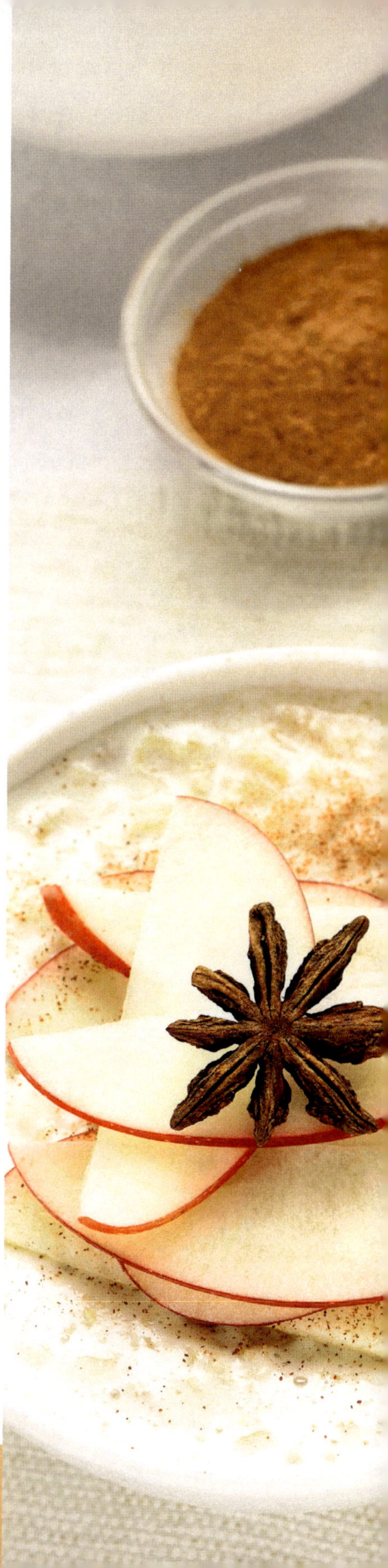

# Western Omelet

**Nutritional Info:**

*Calories: 320 kcal | Carbohydrates: 5.5 g | Protein: 20.5 g | Fat: 24.5 g*
*Total Preparation Time: 20 minutes | Serves: 1*

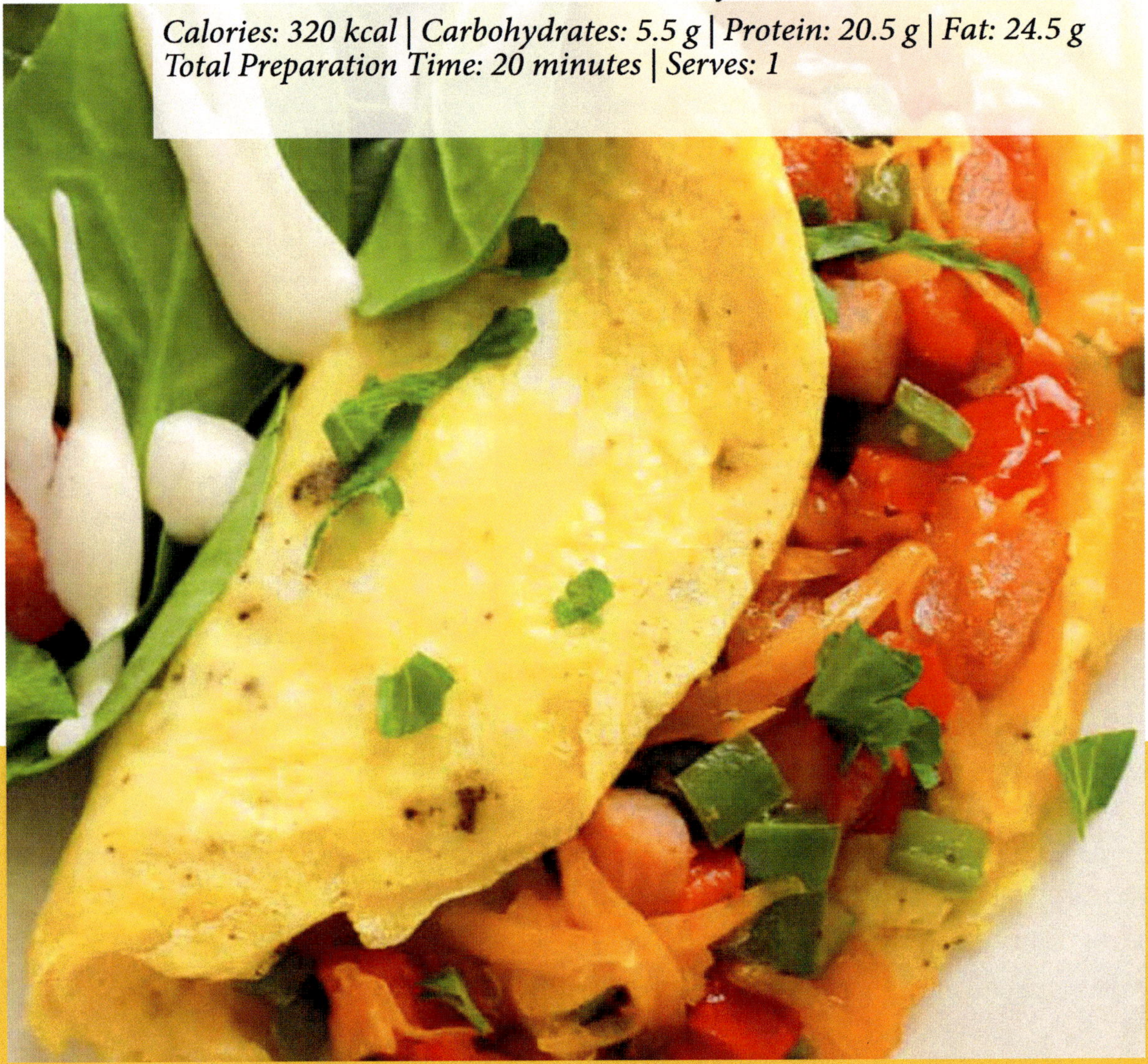

# INGREDIENTS

- *2 medium-sized eggs*
- *2 green onions, sliced*
- *2 tsp. of butter, softened*
- *Salt and black pepper powder, to taste*
- *⅓ cup of fresh mushrooms, diced*
- *4 tbsp. of green bell peppers, diced*
- *4 tbsp. of cooked ham strips (optional)*

# DIRECTIONS

1. Place a small skillet over medium heat.
2. Melt 1 teaspoon of butter.
3. Add mushrooms, bell peppers, and green onions to the skillet.
4. Cook for about 5 minutes, stirring occasionally, until tender.
5. (*Optional*) Stir in the ham and cook for an additional 1 minute, or until heated through.
6. Season with sea salt and freshly ground pepper.
7. Remove the filling mixture from the skillet and transfer it to a small bowl.
8. In a bowl, whisk the eggs.
9. Season the eggs with salt and pepper.
10. Over medium-high heat, preheat the same skillet.
11. Raise the heat to high and then add the remaining 1 teaspoon of butter until it foams— about 30 seconds.
12. Add the eggs to the skillet.
13. Lift the omelet's edges to allow the uncooked egg to run beneath the cooked edges and contact the hot skillet.
14. Shake and tilt the skillet to reposition the raw egg.
15. Repeat for approximately 2 minutes until the top is set, moist, and soft.
16. Distribute the filling evenly over one half of the omelet.
17. Fold the leftover omelet over the filling.
18. Serve and enjoy!

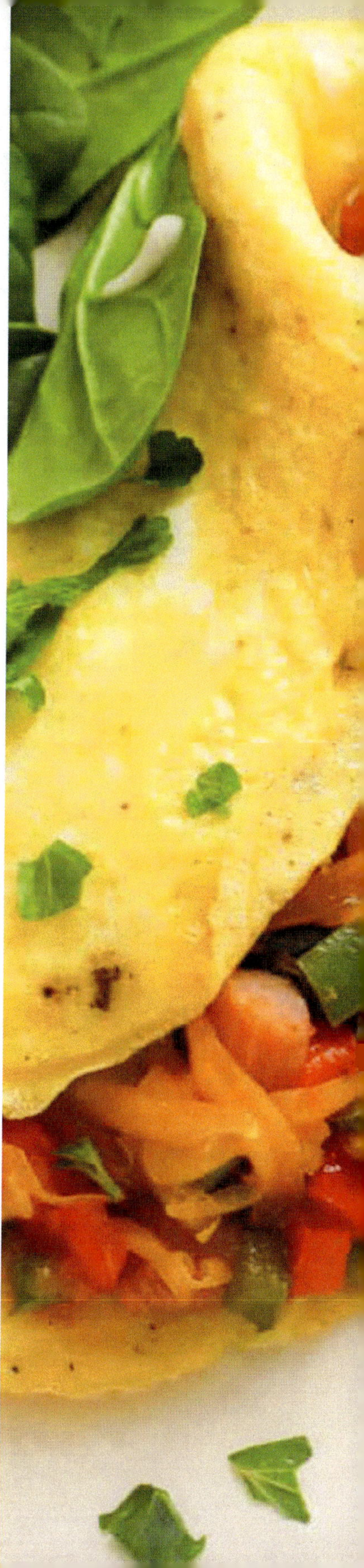

# Ultimate Low-Carb Ham and Cheese Omelet

LOVE'S HOLISTIC NUTRITION

**Nutritional Info:**

*Calories: 725 kcal | Carbohydrates: 10.2 g | Protein: 51.9 g | Fat: 52.9 g*
*Total Preparation Time: 17 minutes | Serves: 2*

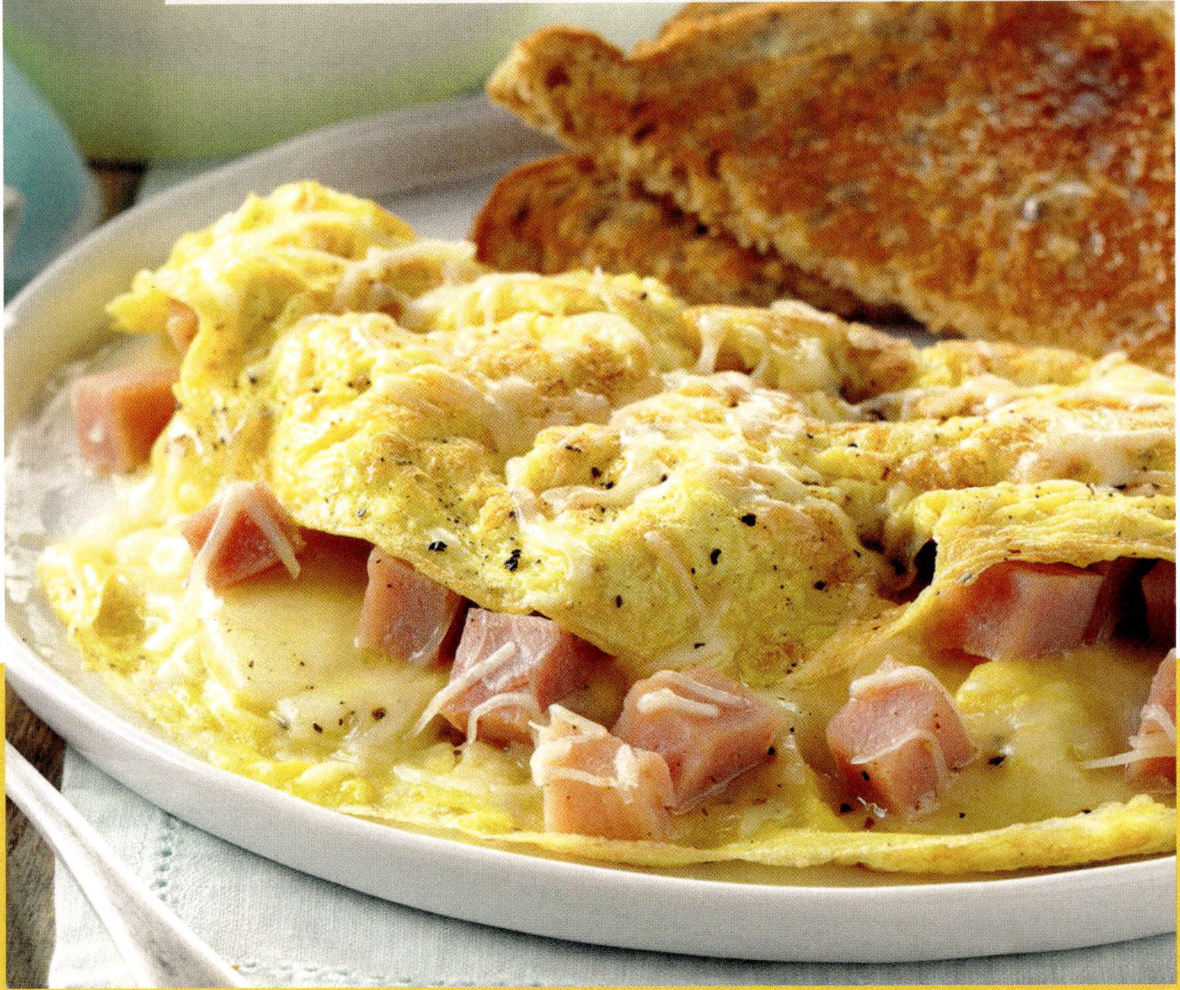

# *INGREDIENTS*

- *2 tbsp. of heavy whipping cream*
- *1 tsp. of salt*
- *½ tsp. of ground black pepper*
- *1 serving of cooking spray*
- *4 oz. of Black Forest ham, diced*
- *¼ cup of green onions, chopped*
- *1 cup of shredded Swiss cheese*
- *5 medium-sized eggs*

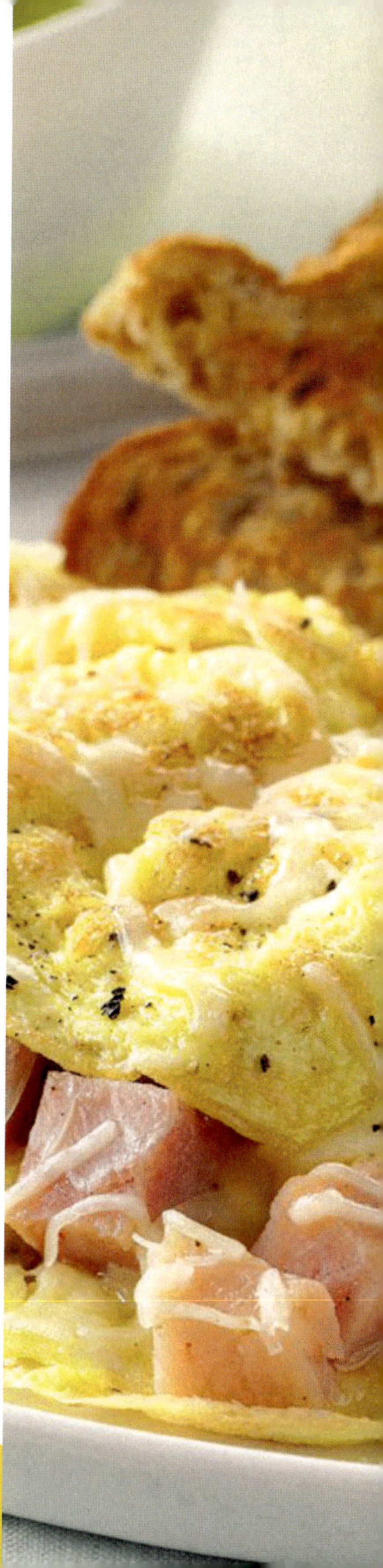

# *DIRECTIONS*

1. Lightly grease a large skillet with cooking spray over medium heat.
2. In a bowl, whisk together the eggs, heavy whipping cream, salt, and pepper.
3. Pour the eggs into the heated skillet, swirling it to coat the bottom of the pan.
4. Cover and cook for approximately 5 minutes, or until the eggs are hard.
5. Sprinkle the shredded cheese, ham, and green onions on the top.
6. Fold one half of the omelet over the fillings and allow it to cook for an additional 2 minutes.
7. Serve and enjoy!

# *Black Bean Breakfast Bowl*

***Nutritional Info*:**

*Calories: 625 kcal | Carbohydrates: 46.6 g | Protein: 27.9 g | Fat: 28.8 g*
*Total Preparation Time: 15 minutes | Serves: 2*

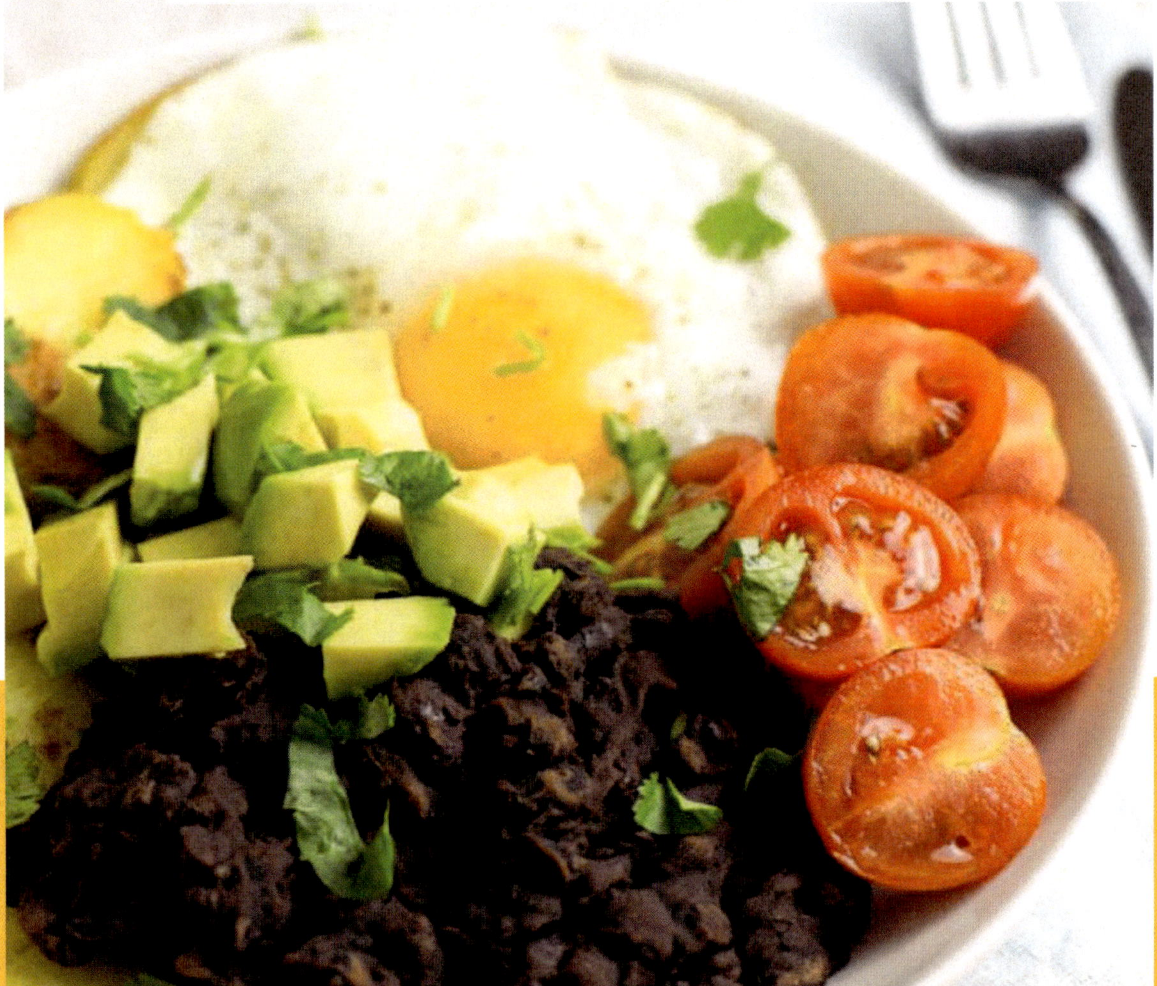

# INGREDIENTS

- *2 tbsp. of olive oil*
- *1 avocado, peeled and chopped*
- *¼ cup of salsa*
- *Salt and black pepper, to taste*
- *4 eggs, lightly beaten*
- *1 can (15 oz) of black beans, drained*

# DIRECTIONS

1. Place a small saucepan over medium heat.
2. Heat the olive oil.
3. Add the eggs to the saucepan.
4. Cook and whisk the eggs for about 3 to 5 minutes, or until they are set.
5. In a microwave-safe bowl, add the black beans and microwave it on the high setting for approximately 1 minute, or until heated.
6. Divide the warmed black beans evenly between 2 serving bowls.
7. Top each bowl with scrambled eggs, avocado, and salsa.
8. Season each bowl with salt and black pepper, to taste.
9. Serve and enjoy!

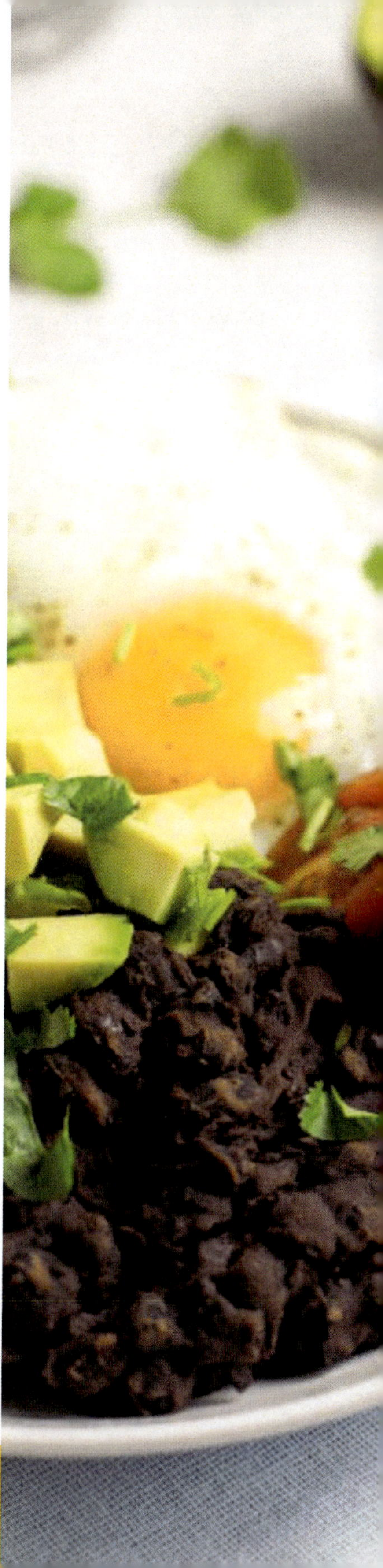

# Breakfast Kidney Beans

**Nutritional Info:**

*Calories: 298 kcal | Carbohydrates: 28.8 g | Protein: 12.5 g | Fat: 11.4 g*
*Total Preparation Time: 40 minutes | Serves: 4*

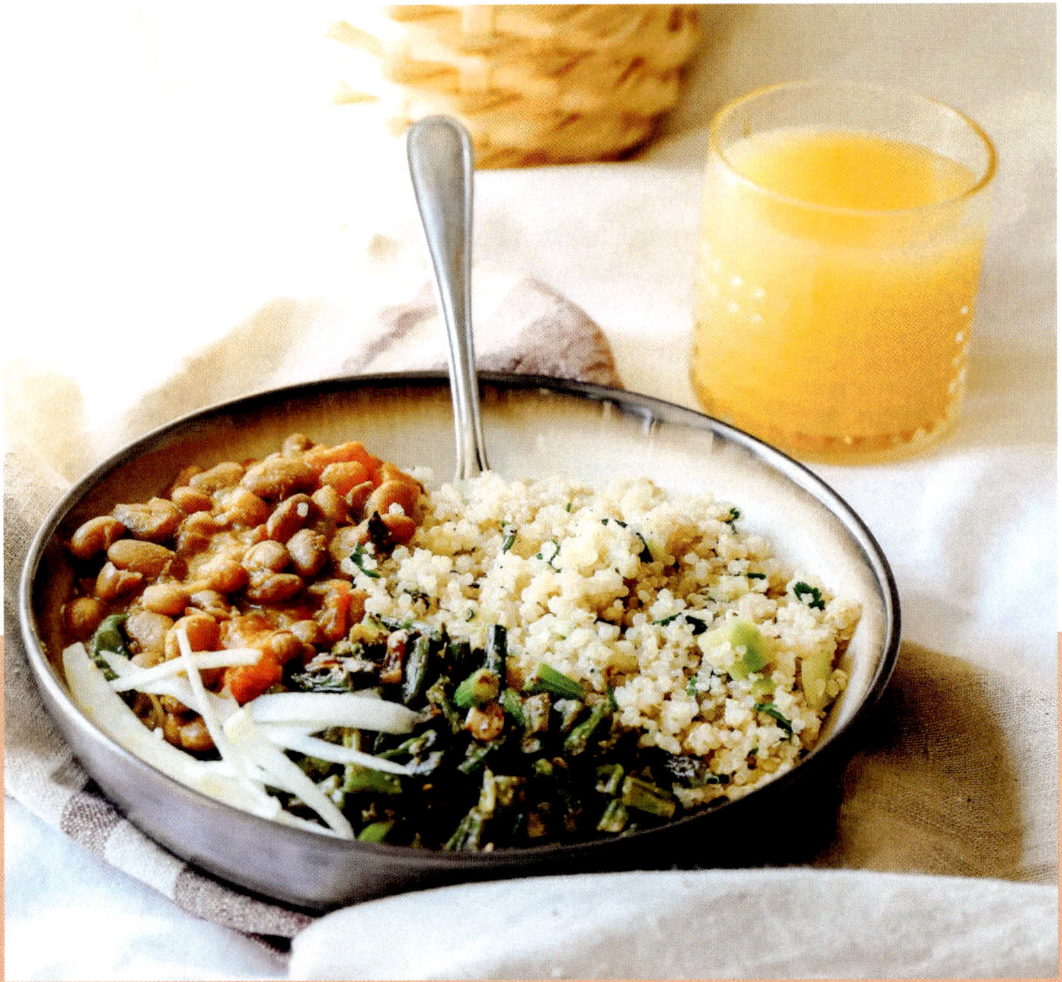

# *INGREDIENTS*

- *3 tbsp. of olive oil*
- *2 small onions, chopped*
- *15 oz. of red kidney beans, undrained*
- *1 large tomato, diced*
- *2 tsp. of tomato paste*
- *Salt and black pepper, to taste*
- *1½ tsp. of ground cumin*
- *1½ tsp. of curry powder*
- *1 jalapeno pepper, finely chopped*

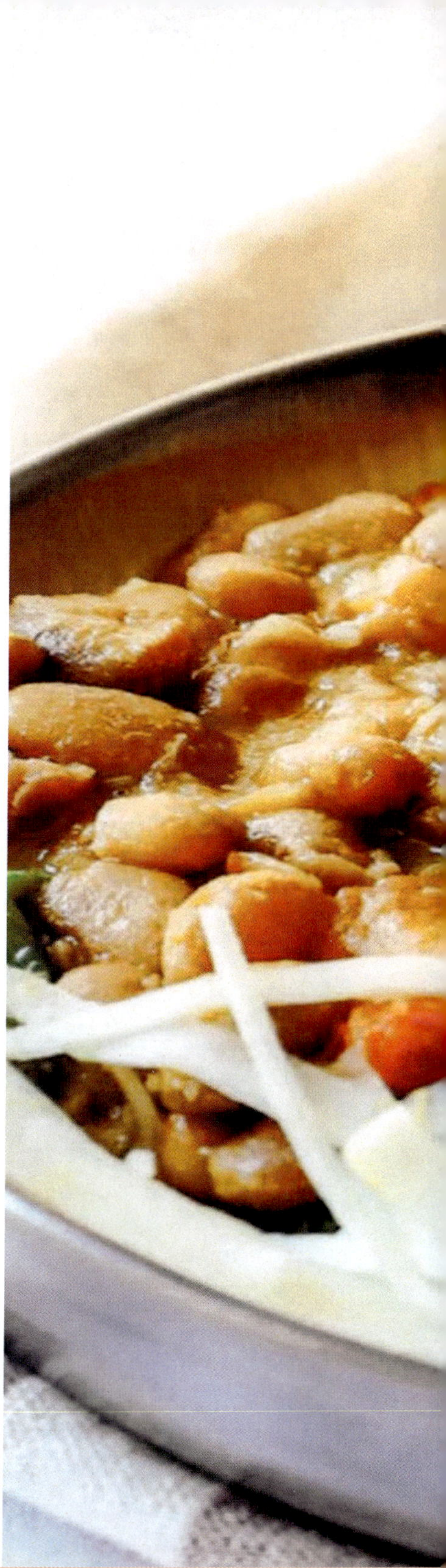

# *DIRECTIONS*

1. Place a large skillet over medium heat.
2. Heat the olive oil.
3. Sauté the onions in the olive oil, frequently turning it until transparent, for about 5 minutes.
4. Stir in the jalapeño pepper and cook it for an additional 5 minutes, or until softened.
5. Combine the tomato and tomato paste with the onions and jalapeno pepper.
6. Pour in the kidney beans and their liquid.
7. Add in the cumin and curry powder.
8. Heat the mixture to a boil.
9. Decrease the heat to medium-low.
10. Simmer for about 15 minutes, until the beans are warmed and the sauce has thickened.
11. Serve and enjoy!

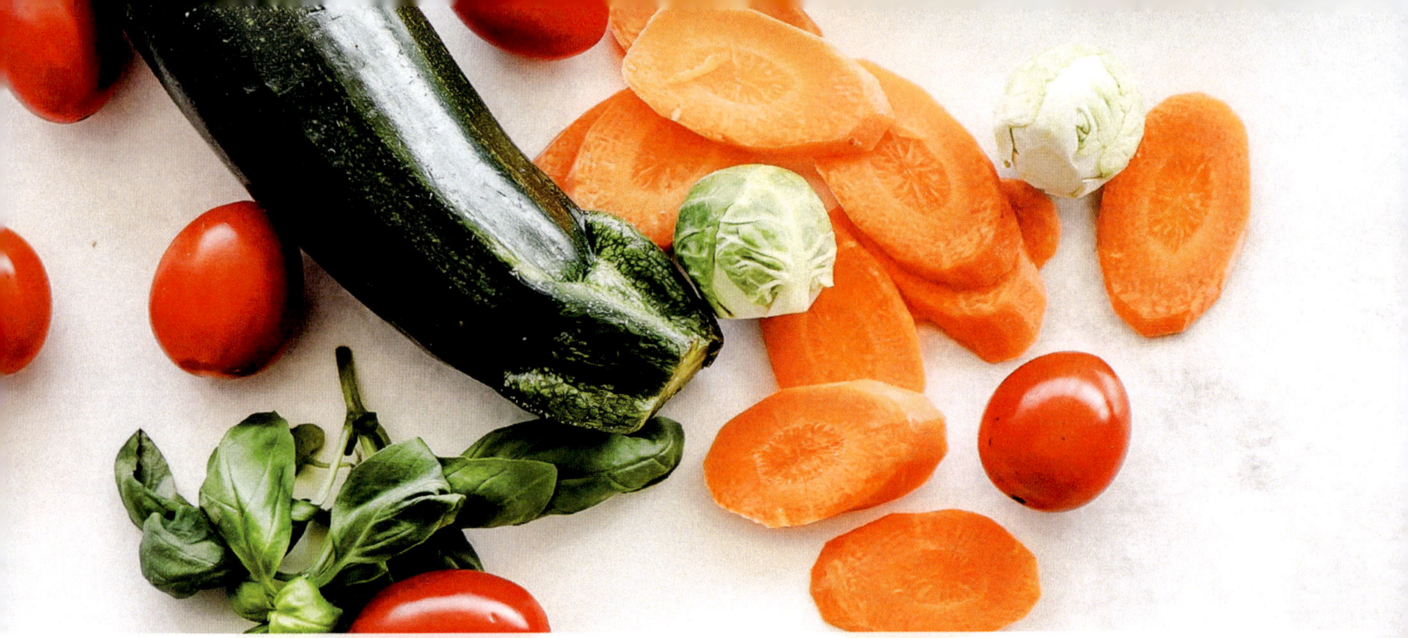

# *Lunch Recipes*

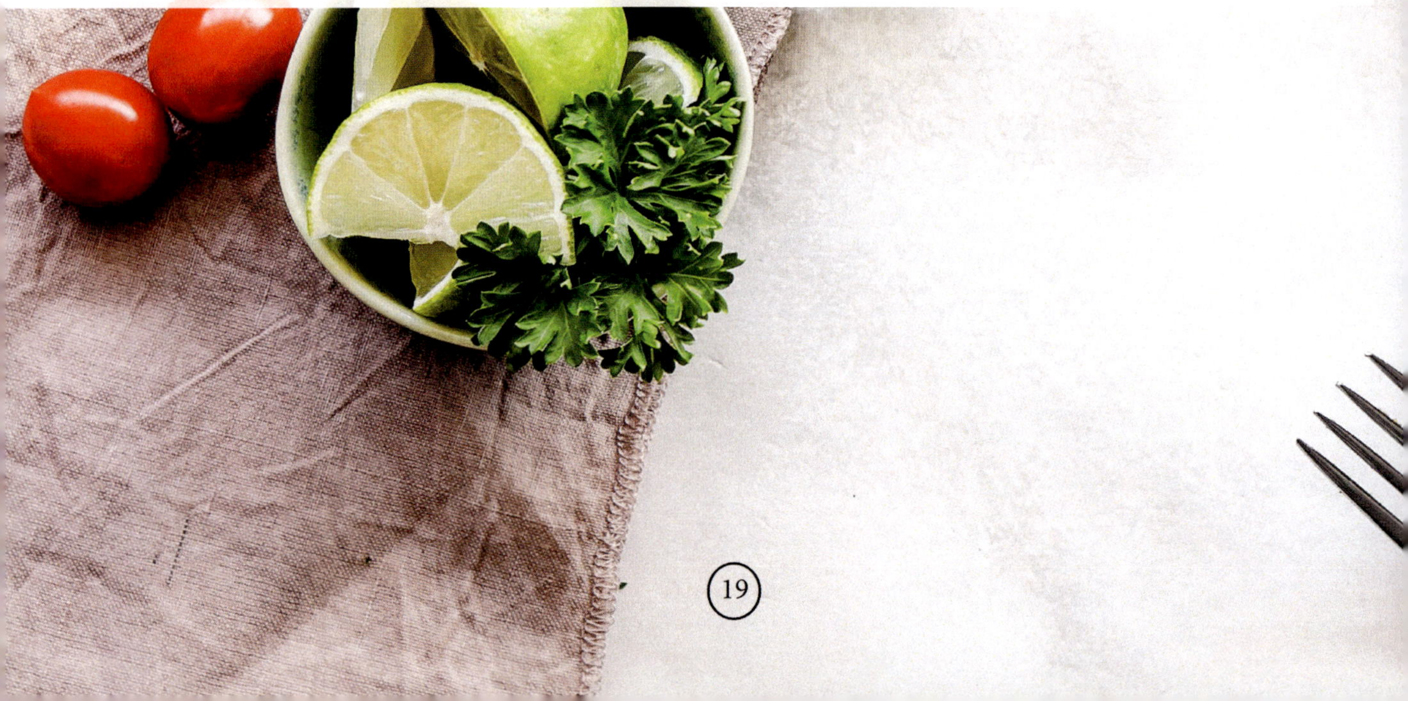

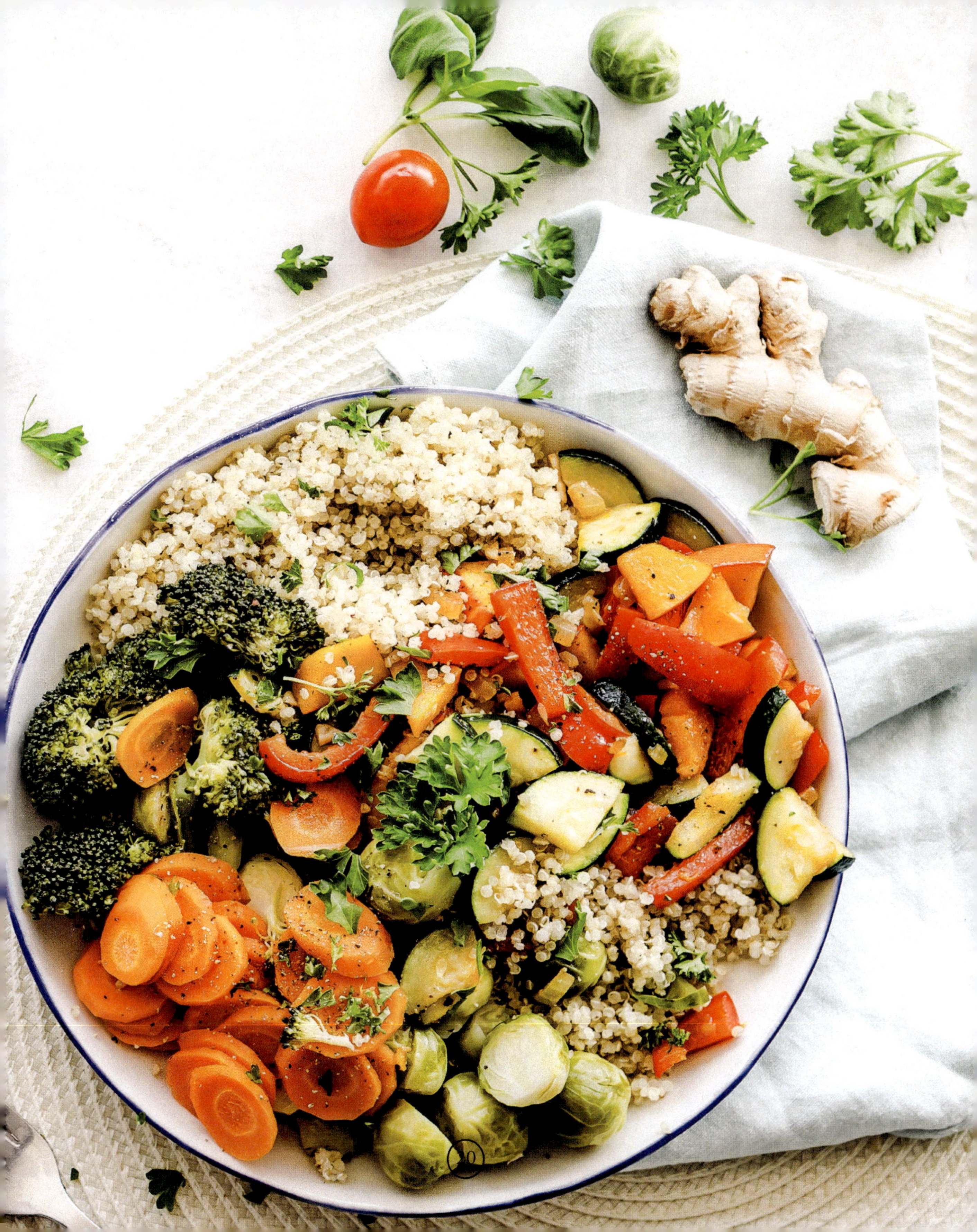

# Mediterranean Pasta Salad

LOVE'S HOLISTIC NUTRITION

**Nutritional Info:**

*Calories: 302 kcal | Carbohydrates: 38 g | Protein: 15 g | Fat: 10 g*
*Total Preparation Time: 15 minutes | Serves: 6-8*

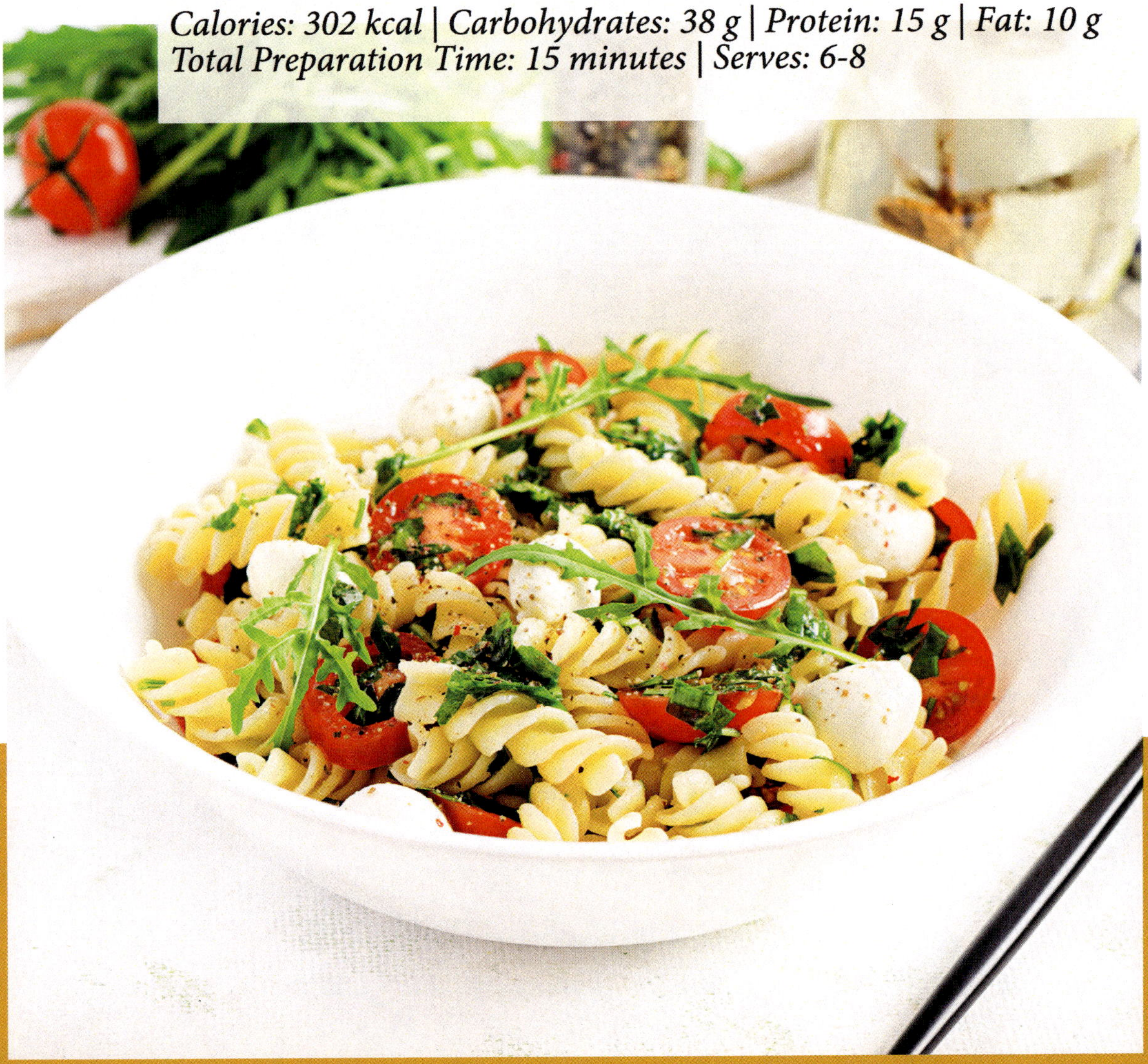

# *INGREDIENTS*

*Mediterranean Pasta Ingredients:*

- *12 oz. of dry pasta*
- *1 medium-sized English cucumber, cubed*
- *1 pint of grape tomatoes, chopped*
- *⅔ cup of Kalamata olives, sliced*
- *4 oz. of feta cheese, crumbled*
- *½ medium-sized red onion, peeled and sliced*

*Lemon-Herb Vinaigrette Ingredients:*

- *4 tbsp. of extra virgin olive oil*
- *3 tbsp. of red wine vinegar*
- *1 tbsp. of freshly squeezed lemon juice*
- *2 tsp. of dried oregano, minced*
- *1 tsp. of honey*
- *2 garlic cloves, minced*
- *¼ tsp. of ground black pepper*
- *¼ tsp. of salt*
- *Pinch of ground red pepper flakes*

# *DIRECTIONS*

To make the vinaigrette:

1. Take the medium-sized bowl and add ingredients to it.
2. Whisk them well until combined.

To make the pasta:

1. In a large stockpot of generously salted water, prepare the pasta according to the packet directions.
2. Rinse the pasta under cold water for approximately 20-30 seconds, or until it is no longer hot.
3. In a large-sized mixing bowl, transfer the pasta.
4. Combine the cucumber, tomatoes, Kalamata olives, feta cheese, and red onion in a mixing bowl.
5. Drizzle all of the vinaigrette over the top, evenly.
6. Toss until the dressing evenly distributed.
7. If desired, garnish with additional feta and black pepper.
8. Serve and enjoy!

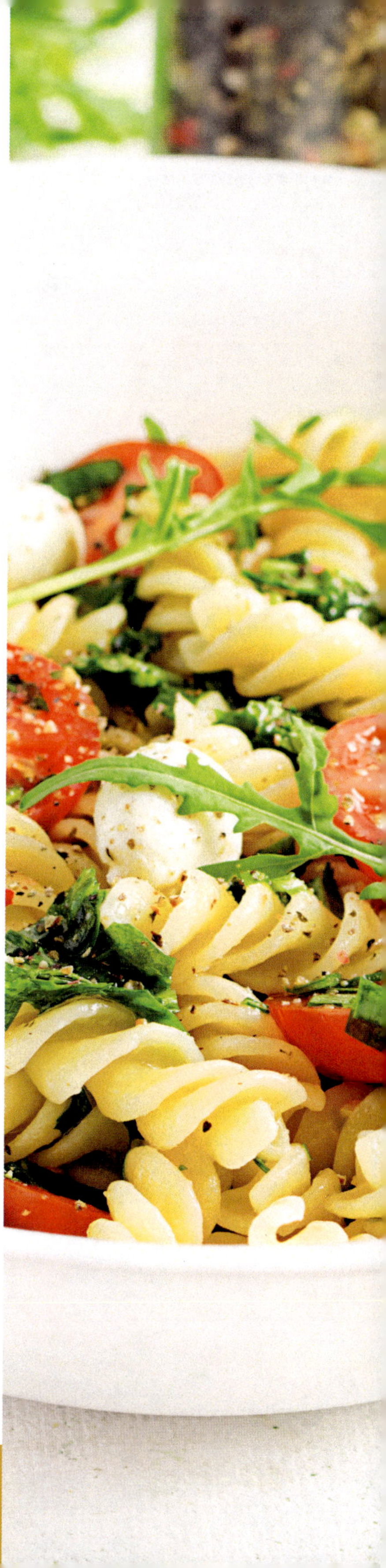

# *Healthy Chicken Salad Recipe*

LOVE'S HOLISTIC NUTRITION

***Nutritional Info:***

*Calories: 361 kcal | Carbohydrates: 23 g | Protein: 20 g | Fat: 21 g*
*Total Preparation Time: 15 minutes | Serves: 4*

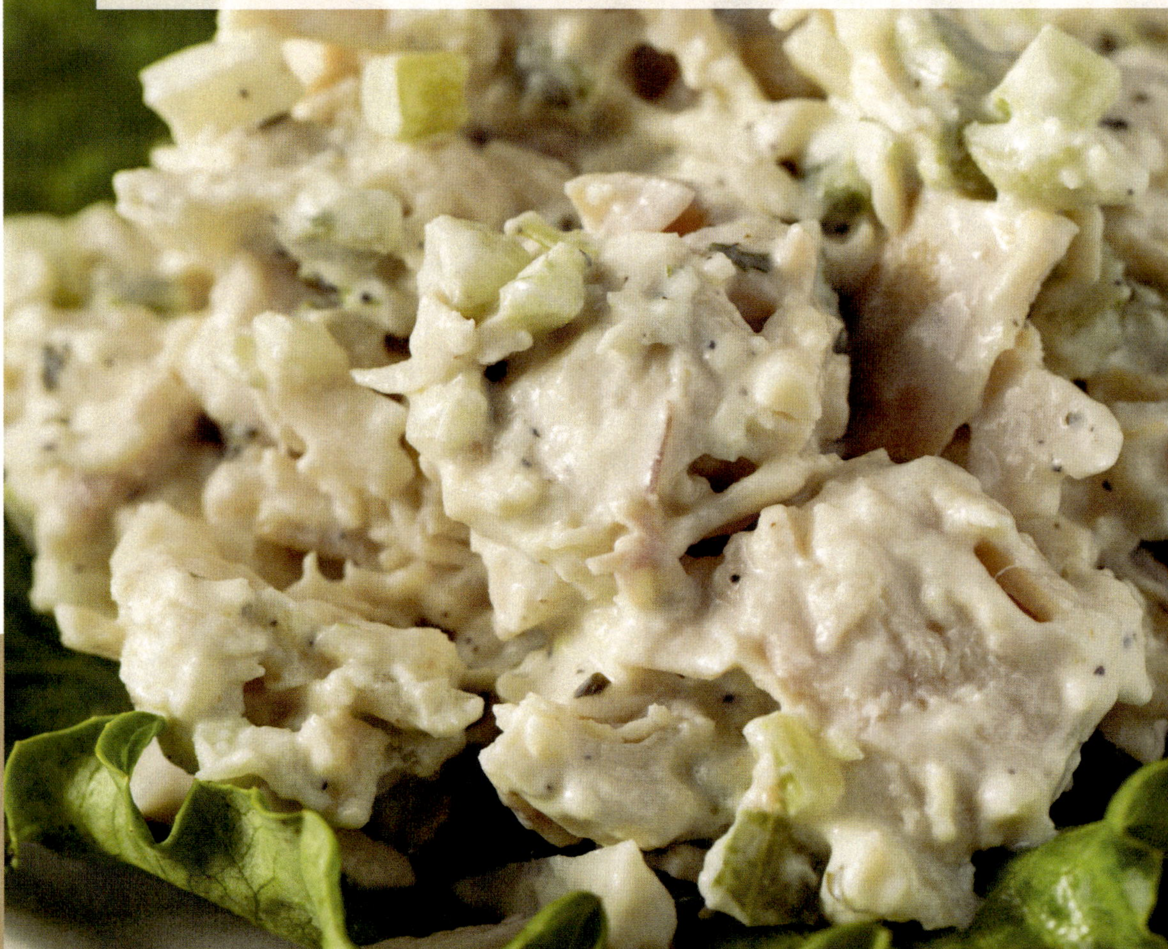

# INGREDIENTS

- *8 cups of Napa cabbage*
- *4 cups (½ head) of red cabbage*
- *½ tbsp. of white sugar*
- *2 cups of cooked chicken, shredded*
- *⅓ cup of Asian-style dressing (or any you like)*
- *1 cup of fresh cilantro leaves, washed and cleaned*
- *1 cup of mandarin oranges (canned), drained*
- *¼ cup of toasted almonds, chopped*
- *Salt and black pepper, according to taste*

# DIRECTIONS

1. Remove the cabbage cores and thinly slice them, lengthwise.
2. Toss in a large basin with sugar.
3. Combine and blend the cabbage, cilantro, mandarin oranges, almonds, and the remaining vinaigrette in a medium bowl.
4. Top with sea salt and freshly ground pepper.
5. Serve and enjoy!

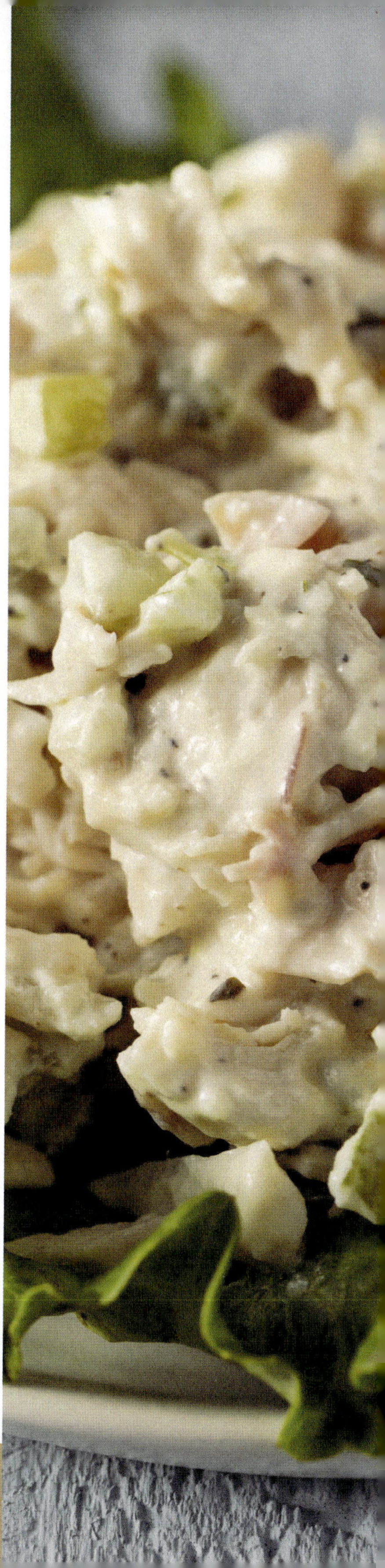

# Creamy Veggie Mac and Cheese

**Nutritional Info:**

*Calories: 243 kcal | Carbohydrates: 35 g | Protein: 10 g | Fat: 7 g*
*Total Preparation Time: 20 minutes | Serves: 2*

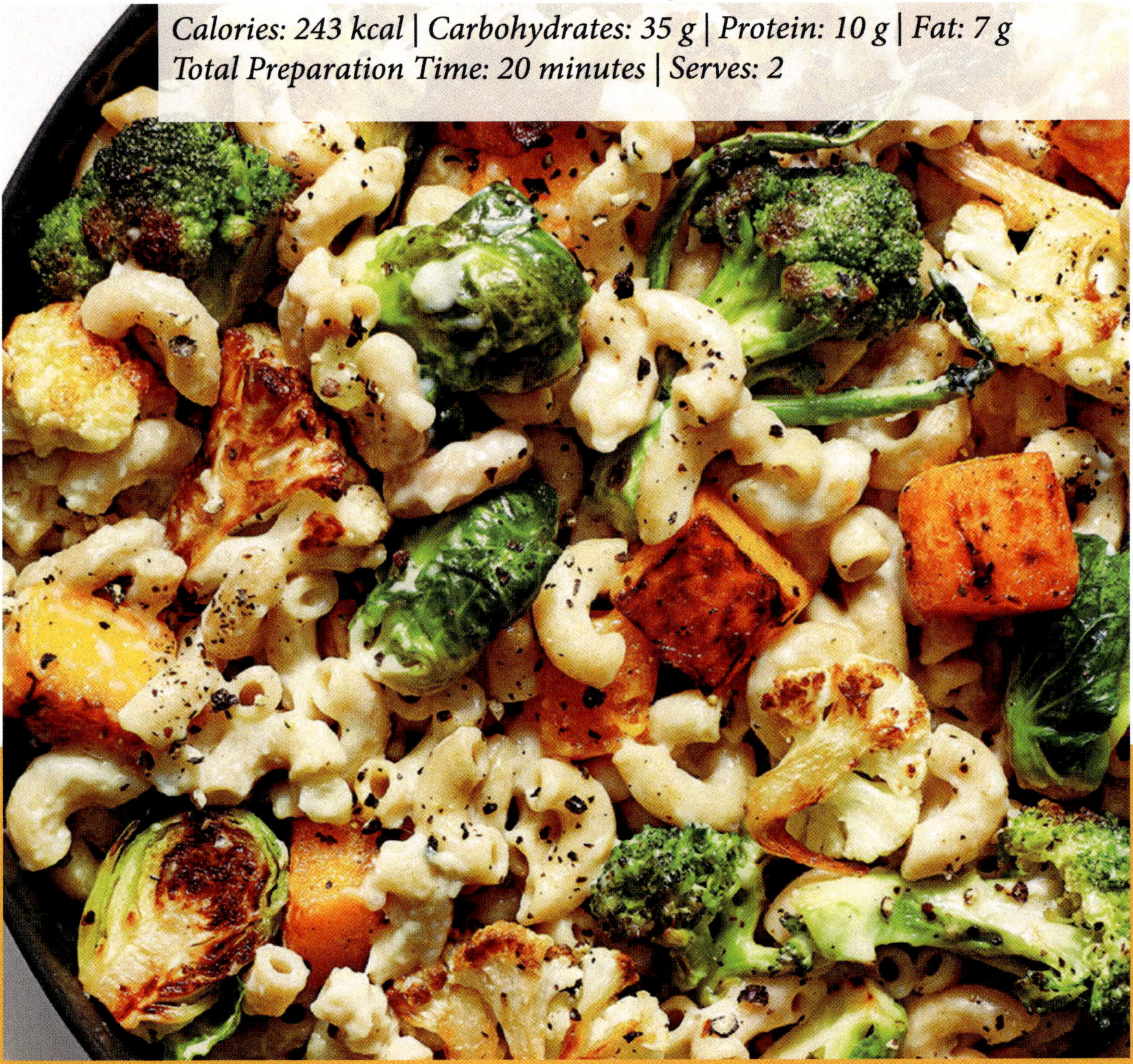

# INGREDIENTS

- *2¾ cups of dried macaroni*
- *1 cup of yellow potatoes, peeled and diced*
- *¼ cup of carrots, peeled and diced*
- *⅓ cup of onion, chopped*
- *¾ cup of water (from the cooked vegetables)*
- *½ cup of raw cashews*
- *¼ cup of coconut milk*
- *2 tbsp. of nutritional yeast flakes*
- *1 tbsp. of lemon juice*
- *1 tsp. of salt, more or less to taste*
- *¼ tsp. of garlic powder*
- *Pinch of cayenne pepper (optional)*
- *Pinch of paprika*

# DIRECTIONS

1. Cook the macaroni noodles al dente, as directed on the package (typically 6-8 minutes in salted water); drain and set aside.
2. In a small boiling pan, bring a few cups of water to a boil.
3. Cook for about 10 minutes, or until the potatoes, carrots, and onions are tender and soft enough to mix. (The cooking time may vary, depending upon the size of the vegetables used.)
4. When the vegetables are tender enough to blend, take them from the cooking water and place them in the blender using a slotted spoon.
5. Add 3/4 cup of the water you boiled the vegetables in, along with the remaining ingredients (including the cashews) to a blender.
6. Blend until smooth.
7. In a serving dish, pour the sauce over the cooked macaroni noodles.
8. Season with salt to taste.
9. Serve and enjoy!

*Additional Option*: Place the pasta mixture in a casserole tray, spread with bread crumbs, and bake for fifteen minutes, or until bread crumbs begin to turn golden brown.

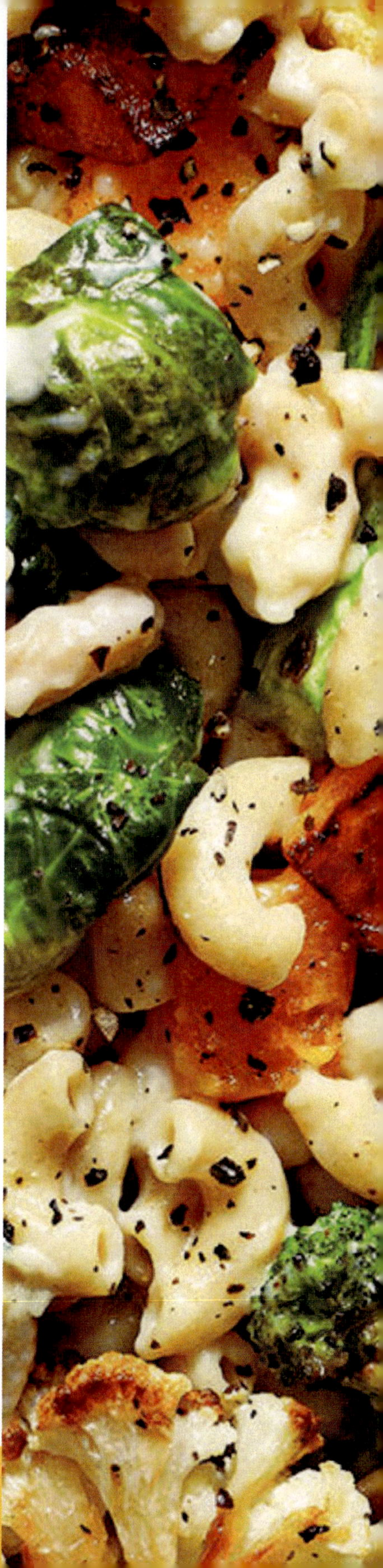

# *Trendy Veggie Pizza*

***Nutritional Info:***

*Calories: 119 kcal | Carbohydrates: 9.5 g | Protein: 3 g | Fat: 0.2 g*
*Total Preparation Time: 40 minutes | Serves: 4*

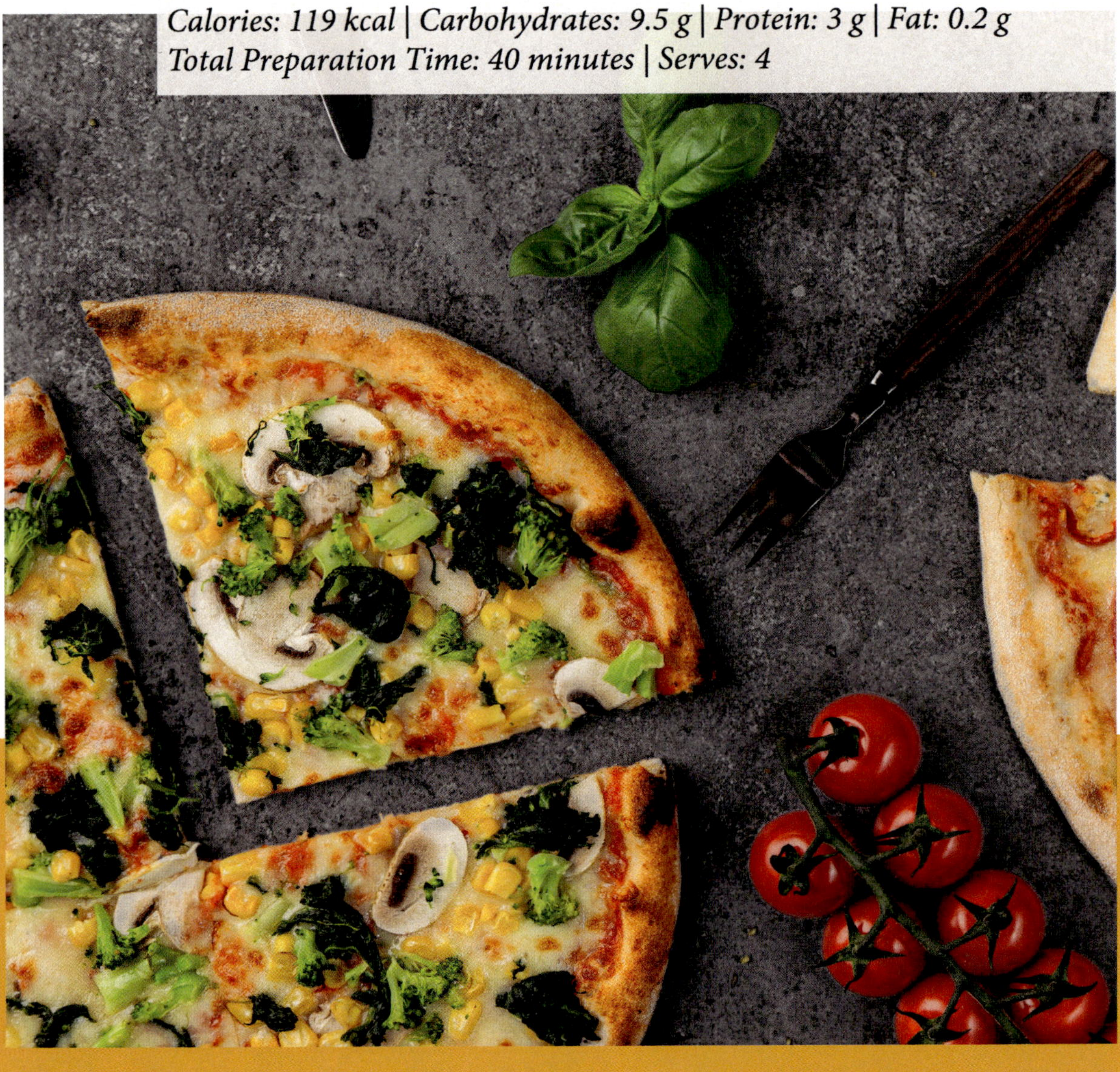

# *INGREDIENTS*

- *450 g of pizza dough, store brought*
- *1 small broccoli, chopped*
- *¼ chopped onion*
- *Cayenne pepper*
- *Canola oil*
- *64 g of fresh basil leaves*
- *2 tbsp. of fresh thyme*
- *Egg-free mayonnaise*
- *Pinch of pepper*
- *Iodized*

# *DIRECTIONS*

1. Preheat the oven to 450° F/ 232° C.
2. In a bowl, combine the broccoli, onion, and cayenne pepper.
3. Coat the mixture with canola oil, salt, and pepper. (The vegetables should be well-seasoned and well-coated.)
4. On a 14-inch pizza pan, stretch the pizza dough.
5. Brush the dough lightly with canola oil and spoon a few scoops of egg-free mayonnaise into the center, spreading it thinly.
6. Distribute the vegetables evenly on the dough.
7. Bake for 15 minutes, or until the crust is browned, and the broccoli is soft and roasted.
8. Remove the pizza from the oven.
9. Top with fresh basil, thyme, and pinches of pepper flakes.
10. Slice, serve, and enjoy!

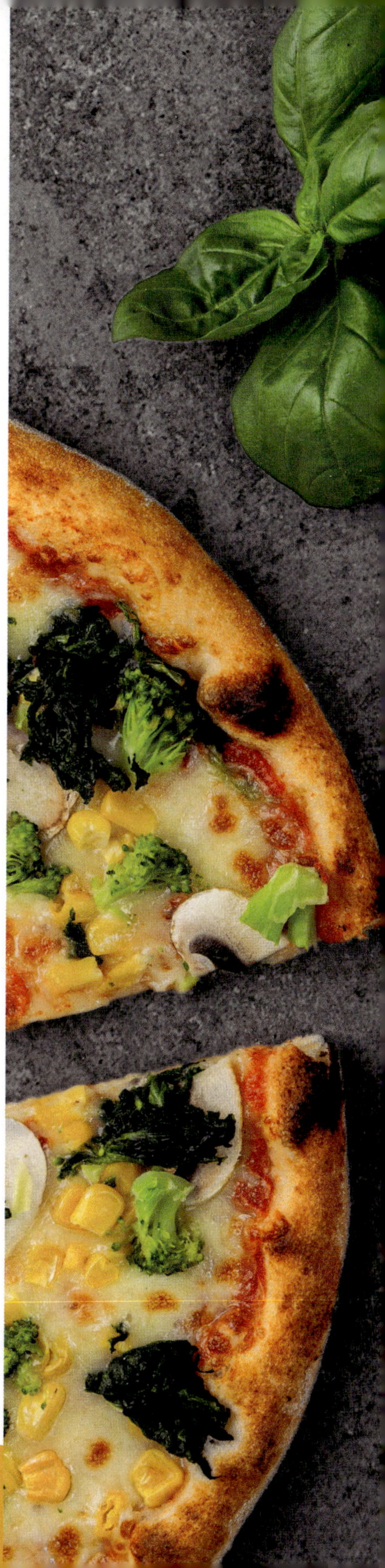

# *Ginger Veggie Stir Fry*

***Nutritional Info:***

*Calories: 119 kcal | Carbohydrates: 9.5 g | Protein: 3 g | Fat: 0.2 g*
*Total Preparation Time: 40 minutes | Serves: 4*

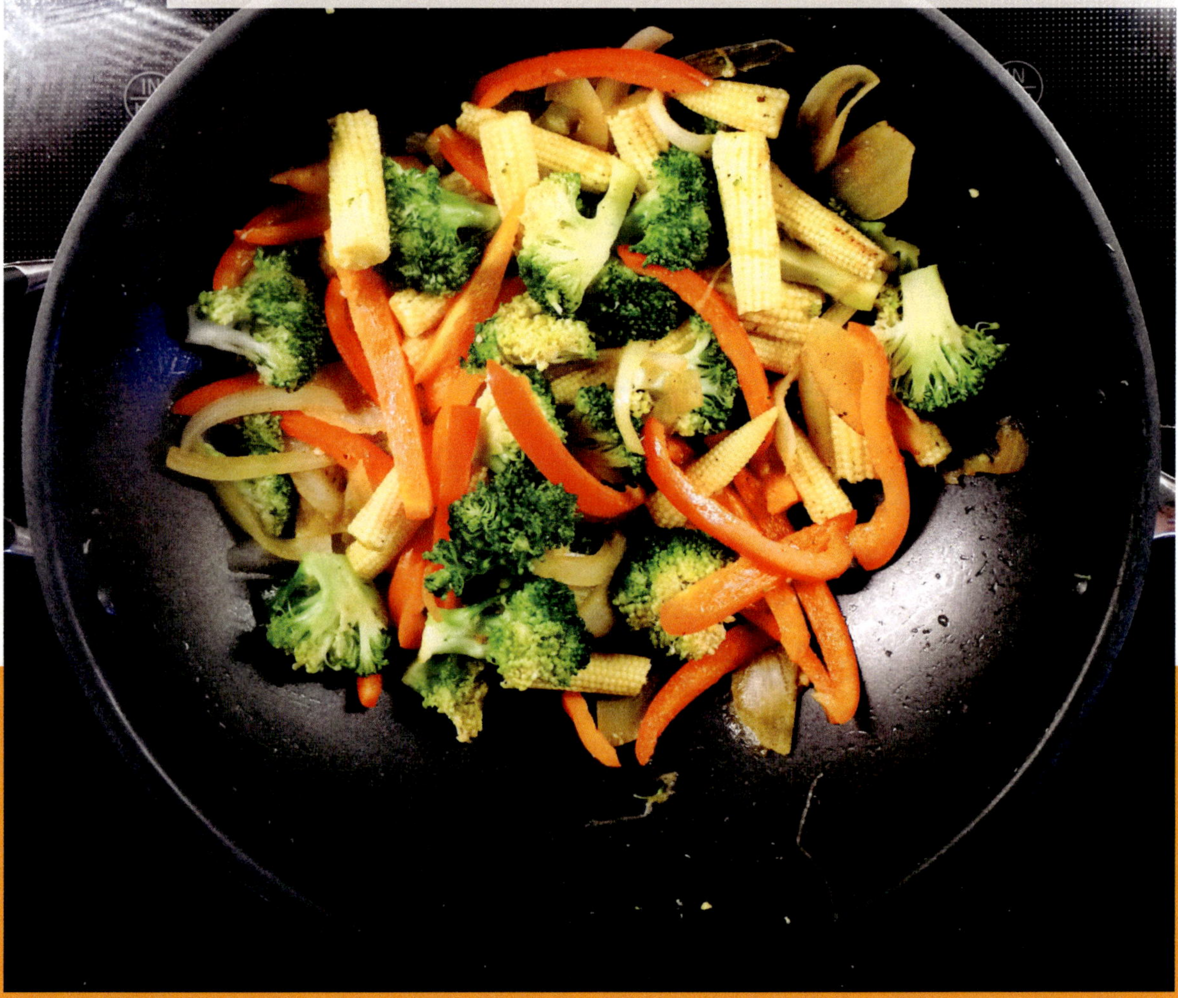

# *INGREDIENTS*

- *1 tbsp. of cornstarch*
- *1 small broccoli, cut into florets*
- *½ cup of snow peas*
- *2 tsp. of fresh ginger roots, chopped*
- *1½ garlic cloves*
- *¼ cup of vegetable oil*
- *½ cup of green beans, halved*
- *¾ cup of carrots*
- *2½ tbsp. of water*
- *¼ cup of onion, chopped*
- *½ tbsp. of salt*
- *2 tbsp. of soy sauce*

# *DIRECTIONS*

1. In a large bowl, mix the cornstarch, garlic, 1 tsp of ginger, and 2 tbsp. of vegetable oil, until the cornstarch is disintegrated.
2. Gently blend in the broccoli, snow peas, carrots, and green beans.
3. Add 2 tbsp. of vegetable oil in a large skillet or wok over medium heat.
4. Cook vegetables in oil for 2 minutes, while mixing continually.
5. Mix in soy sauce and water.
6. Blend in onion, salt, and the leftover 1 tsp. of ginger.
7. Cook until vegetables are delicate, but not mushy.
8. Serve and enjoy!

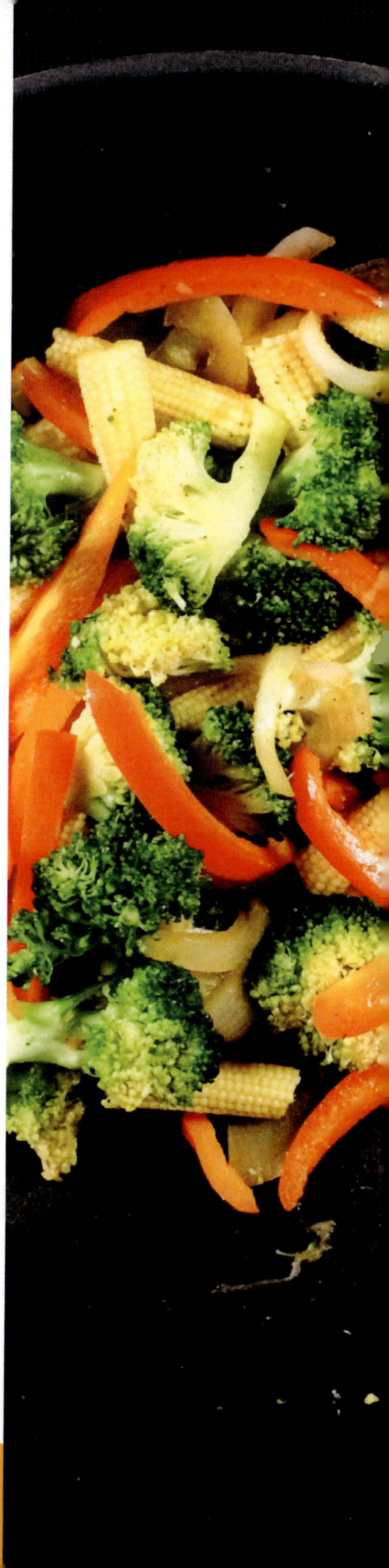

# Honey Walnut Shrimp

**Nutritional Info:**

*Calories: 605 kcal | Carbohydrates: 68 g | Protein: 26.1 g | Fat: 26.3 g*
*Total Preparation Time: 30 minutes | Serves: 4*

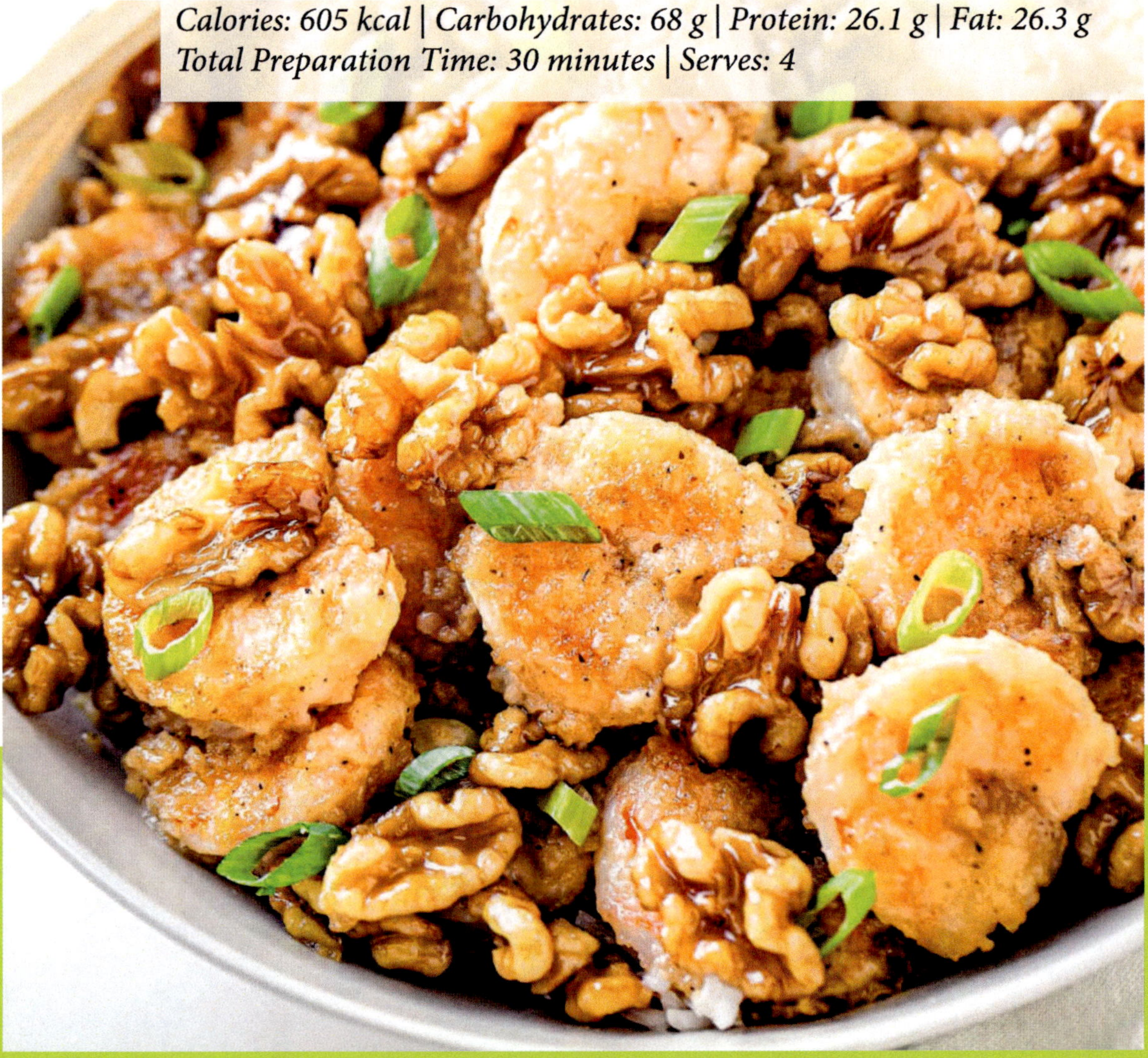

# *INGREDIENTS*

- *⅔ cup of Mochiko Glutinous Rice Flour*
- *¼ cup of mayonnaise*
- *1 lb. of large shrimp, peeled and deveined*
- *4 egg whites*
- *⅔ cup of white sugar*
- *6 tsp. of honey*
- *3 tsp. of canned sweetened condensed milk*
- *½ cup of walnuts*
- *1 cup of water*
- *1 cup of vegetable oil for frying*

# *DIRECTIONS*

1. Place the small saucepan over heat.
2. Add the water and sugar to the saucepan.
3. When the mixture boils, add the walnuts.
4. Allow the walnuts to boil for 2 minutes.
5. Drain and spread the walnuts out on a cookie sheet.
6. In a medium bowl, pulse the egg whites until frothy.
7. Add the rice flour and stir until it's a pasty consistency.
8. Place a deep skillet over medium-high heat with oil.
9. Coat the shrimp in the rice flour batter.
10. Fry the shrimp for about 5 minutes, until golden brown.
11. Remove the shrimp and drain with paper towels.
12. Combine the mayonnaise, honey, and sweetened condensed milk in a medium serving bowl.
13. Toss shrimp in the sauce to coat.
14. Add the candied walnuts on top.
15. Serve and enjoy!

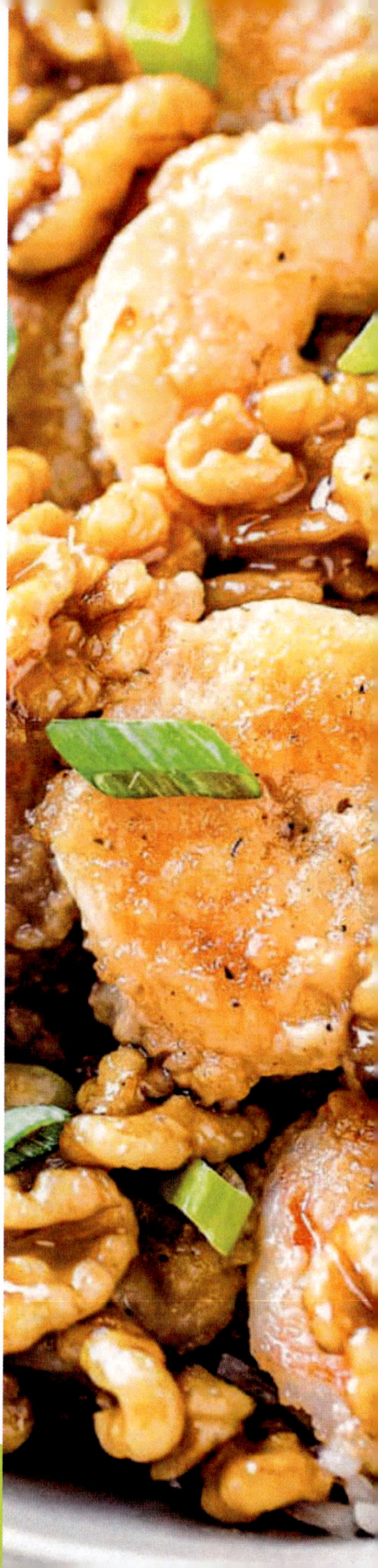

# Grilled Garlic and Herb Shrimp

**Nutritional Info:**

*Calories: 336 kcal | Carbohydrates: 10.2 g | Protein: 37.8 g | Fat: 15.7 g*
*Total Preparation Time: 2 hr, 15 minutes | Serves: 4*

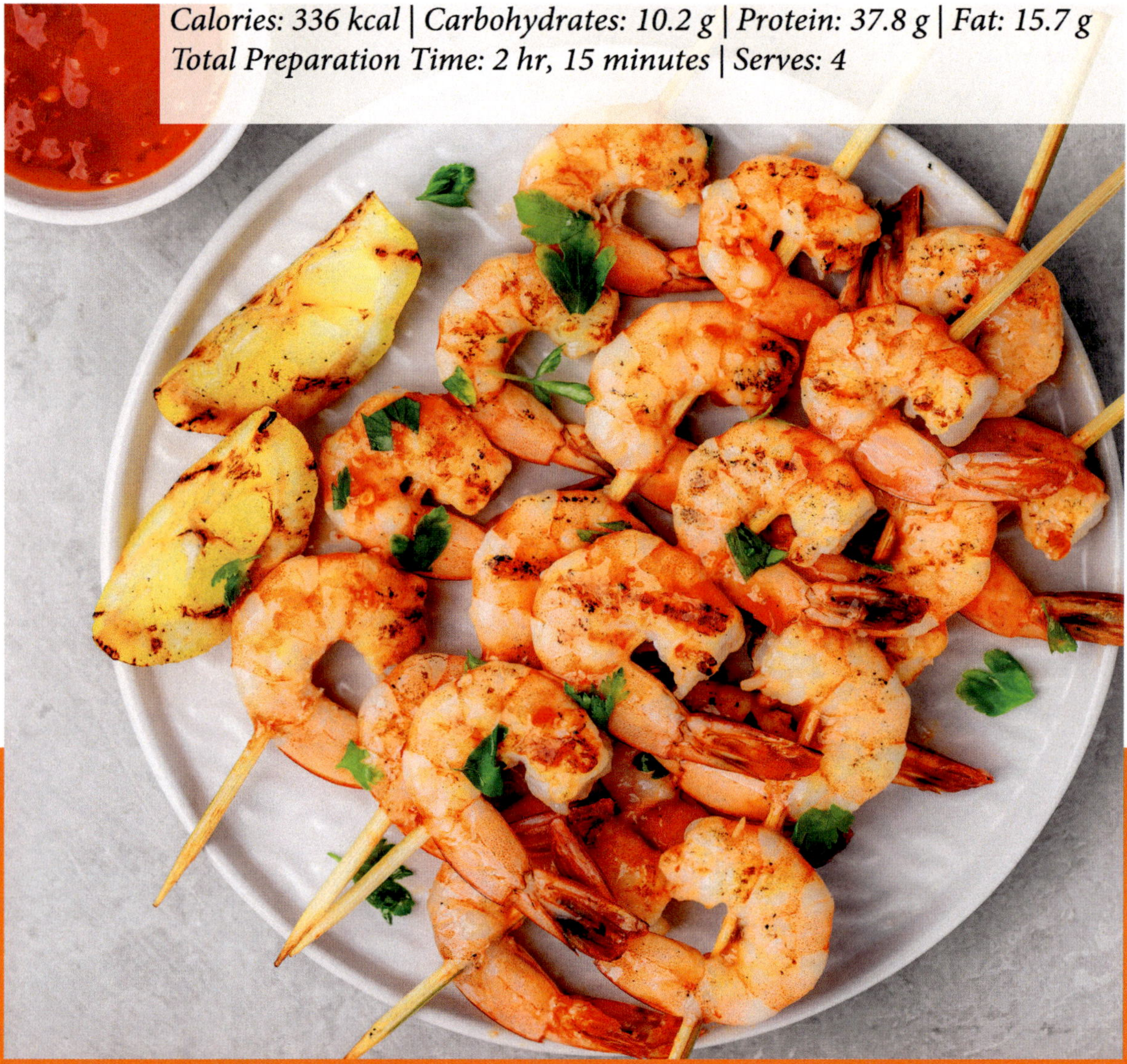

## *INGREDIENTS*

- *2 tsp. of ground paprika*
- *2 tbsp. of fresh minced garlic*
- *2 tsp. of Italian seasoning*
- *2 tbsp. of fresh lemon juice*
- *½ tsp. of ground black pepper*
- *2 tsp. of dried basil leaves*
- *2 tbsp. of brown sugar, packed*
- *2 lb. of large shrimp, peeled and deveined*
- *¼ cup of olive oil*

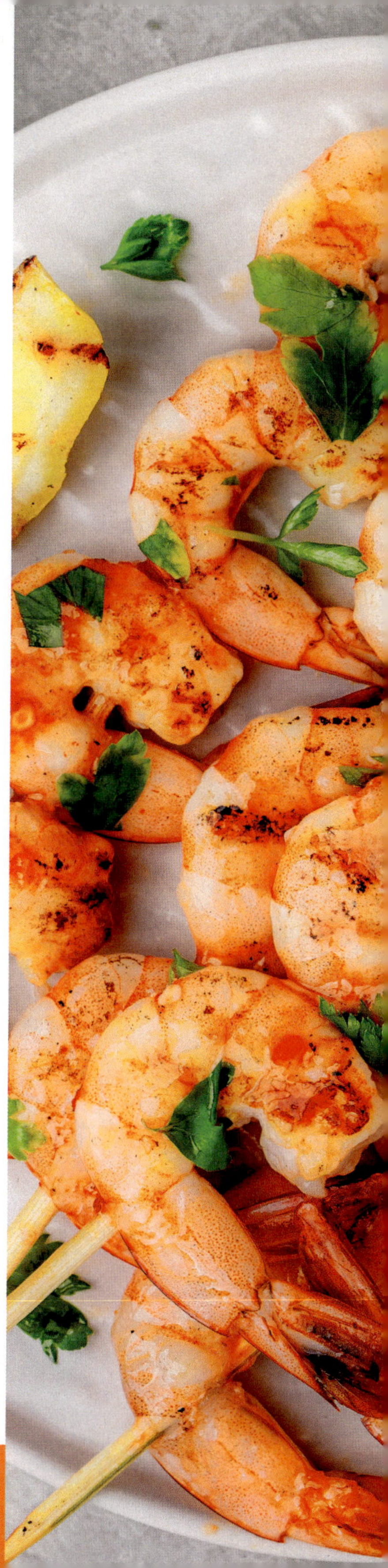

## *DIRECTIONS*

1. In a bowl, whisk together the paprika, garlic, Italian seasoning, lemon juice, olive oil, pepper, basil, and brown sugar, until well combined.
2. Add the shrimp and coat it evenly within the marinade.
3. Cover and refrigerate for at least 2 hours, turning once.
4. Preheat the grill's temperature to medium-high.
5. Lightly oil the grill grate and position it approximately 4 inches away from the heat source.
6. Drain excess marinade from shrimp.
7. Place the shrimp on the grill.
8. Grill the shrimp for 5 to 6 minutes, while flipping.
9. Cook until the shrimp are opaque in the center.
10. Serve right away and enjoy!

# Bacon Sweet Potato Cornbread

**Nutritional Info:**

*Calories: 207 kcal | Carbohydrates: 29.4 g | Protein: 8.7 g | Fat: 5.7 g*
*Total Preparation Time: 55 minutes | Serves: 6*

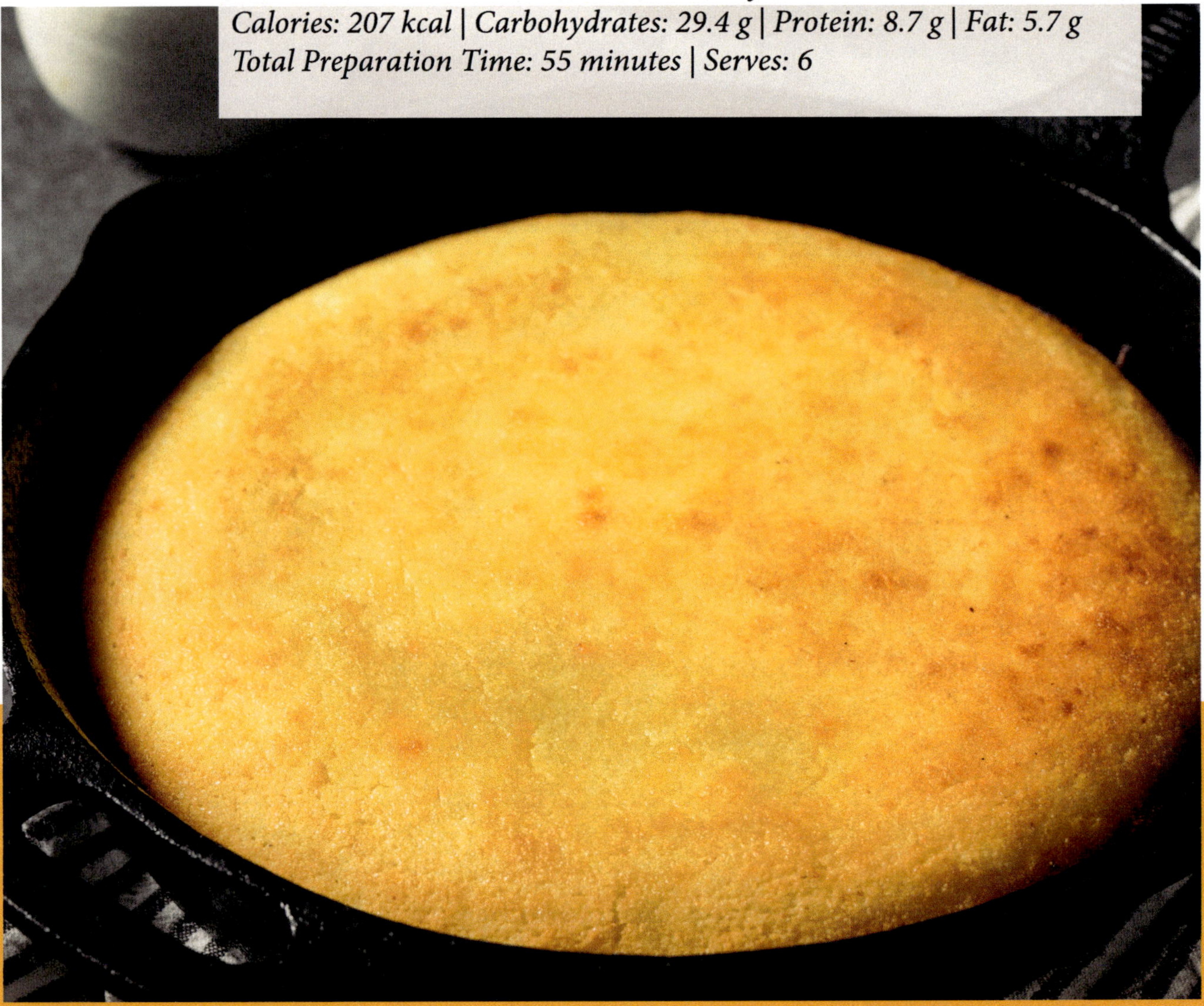

# *INGREDIENTS*

- *1 tsp. of salt*
- *½ tsp. of baking soda*
- *1¼ cups of cornmeal*
- *1 cup of soft buttermilk*
- *5 bacon slices*
- *2 eggs, lightly whisked*
- *1 cup of mashed cooked sweet potatoes*

# *DIRECTIONS*

1. Preheat the oven to 450°F (230°C).
2. In a 9-inch cast-iron skillet over medium-high heat, cook and stir bacon until browned (about 10 minutes).
3. Remove and chop bacon, reserving 1 tablespoon of bacon drippings in the skillet.
4. In a bowl, whisk together the cornmeal, salt, and baking soda.
5. In a separate dish, whisk together the sweet potato, buttermilk, and eggs until well blended.
6. Combine the sweet potato mixture and dry ingredients in a large mixing bowl.
7. Add the chopped bacon to the batter.
8. Fill the cast-iron skillet halfway with batter.
9. Bake the cornbread in the preheated oven for about 30 minutes, or until golden, when the bread feels firm.
10. Transfer the cornbread to a serving platter and cut it into wedges.
11. Serve and enjoy!

# *Russian Potato Salad*

**Nutritional Info:**

*Calories: 478 kcal | Carbohydrates: 43.2 g | Protein: 14.8 g | Fat: 28.3 g*
*Total Preparation Time: 50 minutes | Serves: 10*

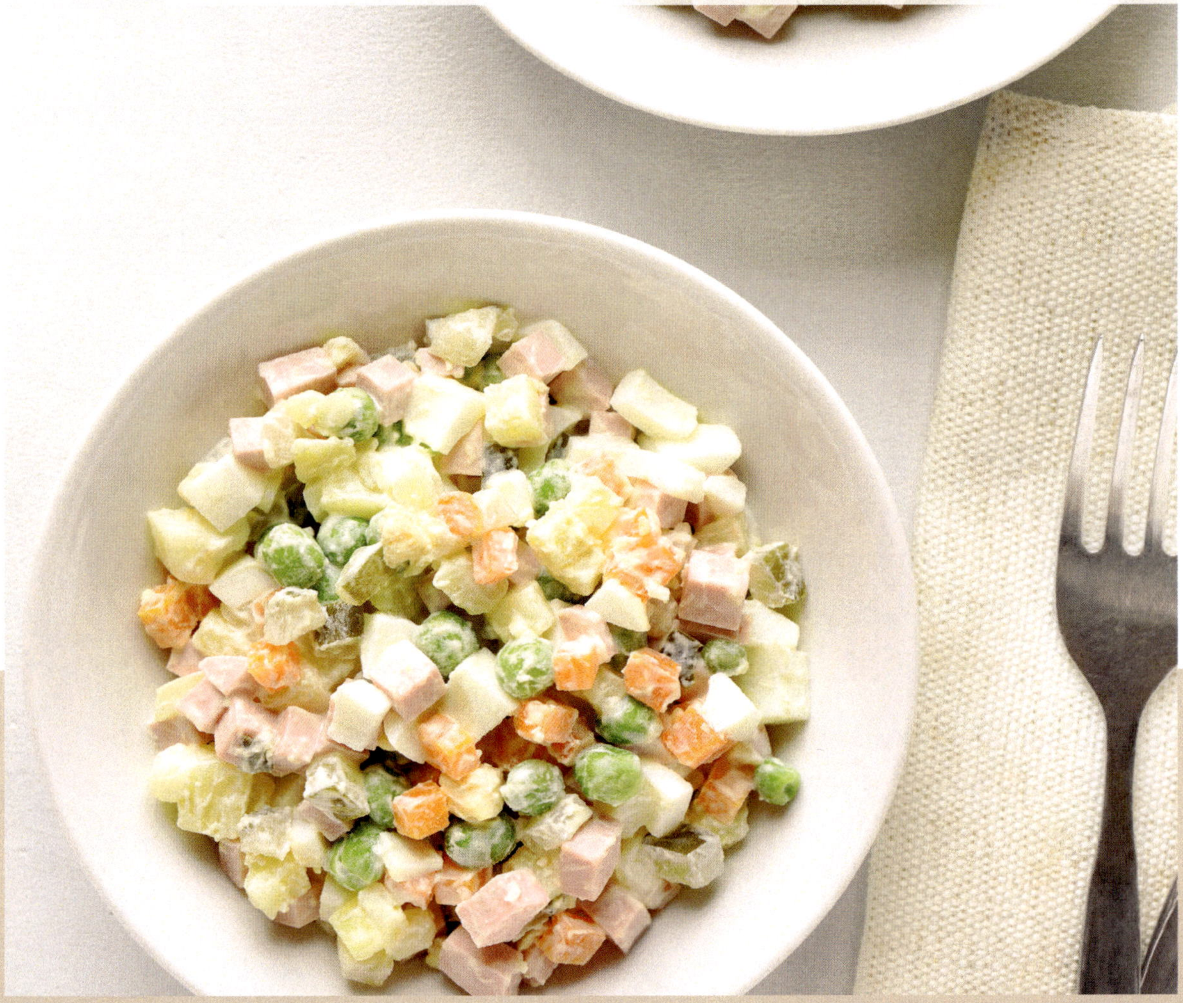

# INGREDIENTS

- *10 small potatoes*
- *1 cup of vegan mayonnaise, any brand*
- *16 oz. package of turkey hot dogs*
- *5 eggs*
- *10 small dill pickles, diced*
- *1 bunch of green onions, chopped*
- *Salt, to taste*
- *15 oz. can of baby peas, drained*

# DIRECTIONS

1. Fill the large pot halfway with water.
2. Add the potatoes.
3. Bring to a boil and cook for about 20 minutes, or until a fork can be easily inserted and removed.
4. Drain and set aside to cool slightly.
5. Boil the hot dogs and eggs for 10 minutes.
6. Drain and put aside to cool.
7. Peel and chop the potatoes.
8. Slice the hot dogs.
9. Gather all ingredients in the large mixing bowl, including the pickles, onions, and peas.
10. Peel the eggs and grate on top of the salad.
11. Top with mayonnaise and salt.
12. Serve and enjoy!

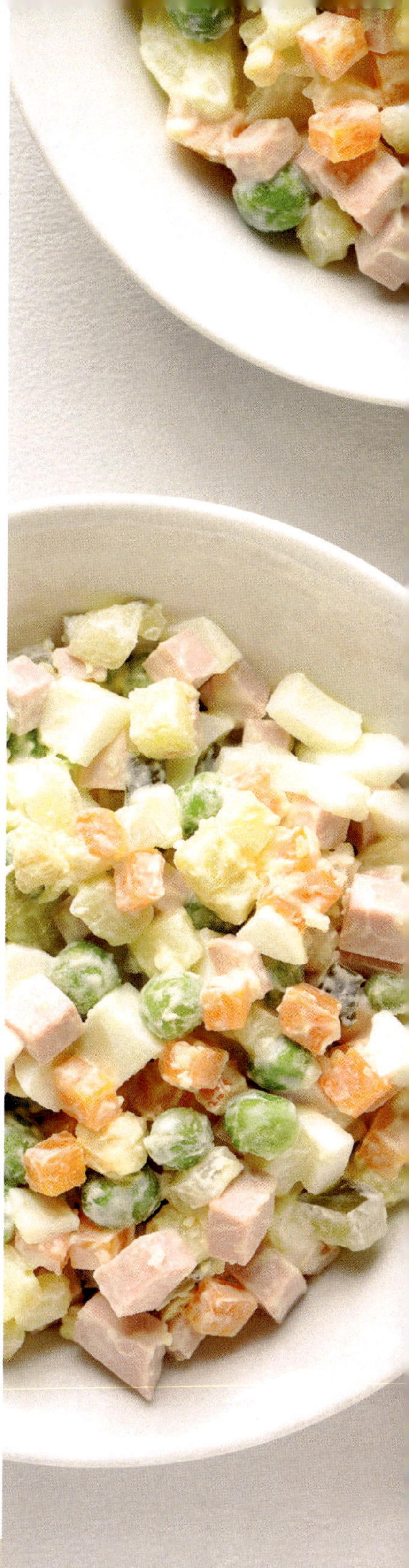

# Cheesy Broccoli Casserole

**Nutritional Info:**
*Calories: 270 kcal | Carbohydrates: 20 g | Fat: 16 g | Protein: 10 g*
*Total Preparation Time: 1 hour, 20 minutes | Serves: 10*

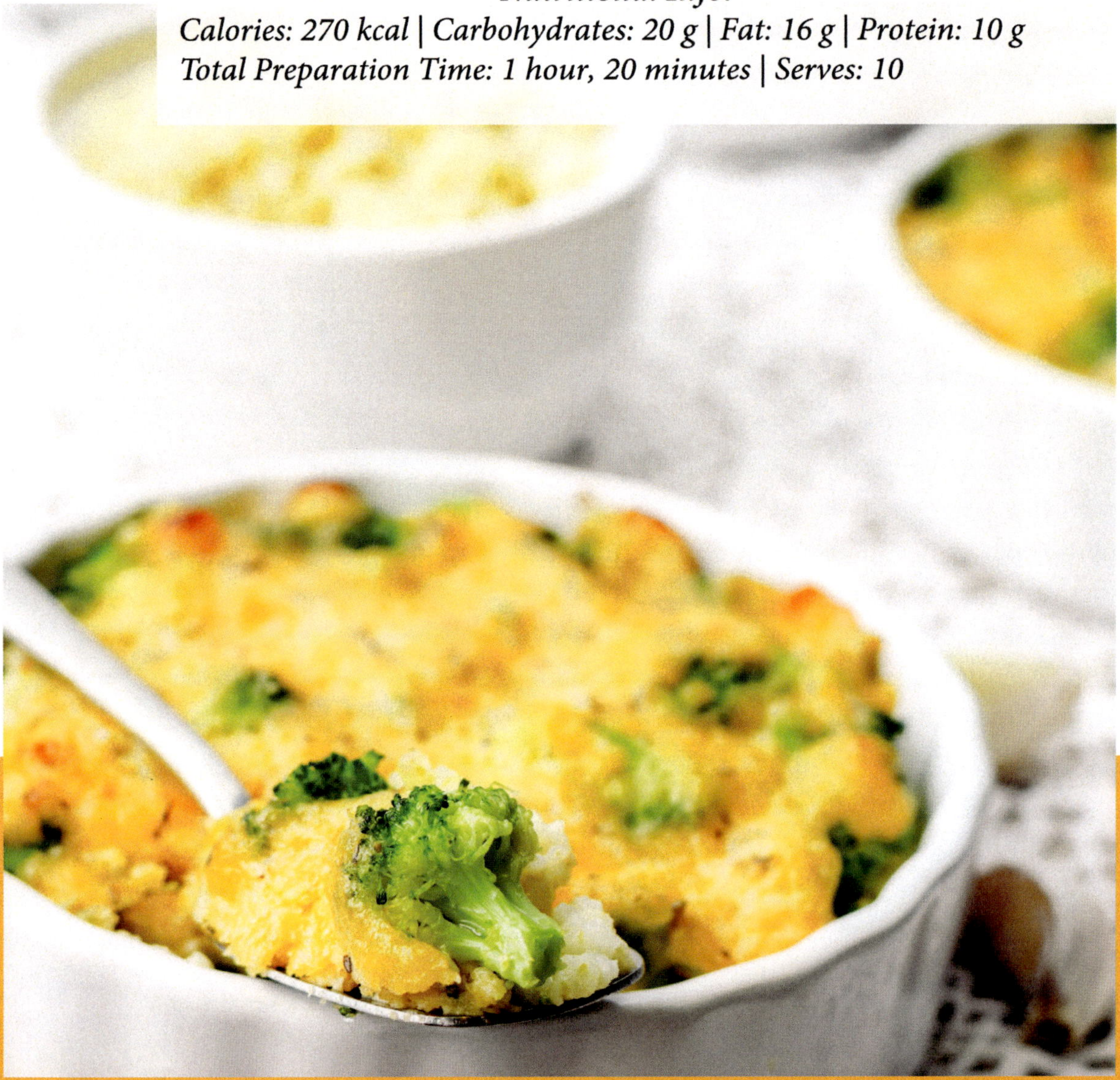

# INGREDIENTS

- *Cooking spray or cooking oil*
- *1 large egg*
- *16 oz. bag of frozen cut broccoli*
- *1 (10¾ oz) can of condensed cream of mushroom soup*
- *6 oz. of Cabot Adirondack Cheddar*
- *½ cup of mayonnaise*
- *1 small onion, chopped*
- *1 sleeve of Ritz crackers, crushed*
- *1 stick (about ½ cup) of Cabot Salted Butter*

# DIRECTIONS

1. Preheat the oven to 350°F.
2. Coat a 9x13 inch baking dish lightly with nonstick cooking spray.
3. In a large mixing bowl, beat the egg with a fork until entirely blended.
4. Add the broccoli, soup, cheese, mayonnaise, and onion, stirring well.
5. Evenly distribute ingredients in a prepared baking dish or pan.
6. Combine the crackers and butter in a small bowl.
7. Sprinkle evenly over the broccoli mixture.
8. Bake for 45 minutes to 1 hour, or until golden and bubbly.
9. Serve and enjoy!

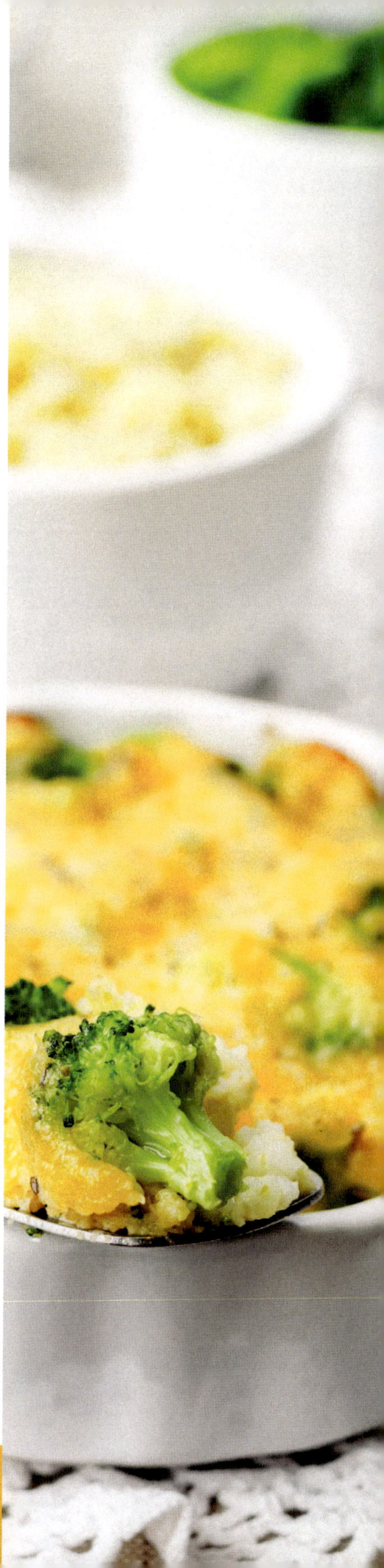

# Cedar Planked Salmon

**Nutritional Info:**

*Calories: 678 kcal | Carbohydrates: 1.7 g | Protein: 61.3 g | Fat: 45.8 g*
*Total Preparation Time: 35 minutes | Serves: 6*

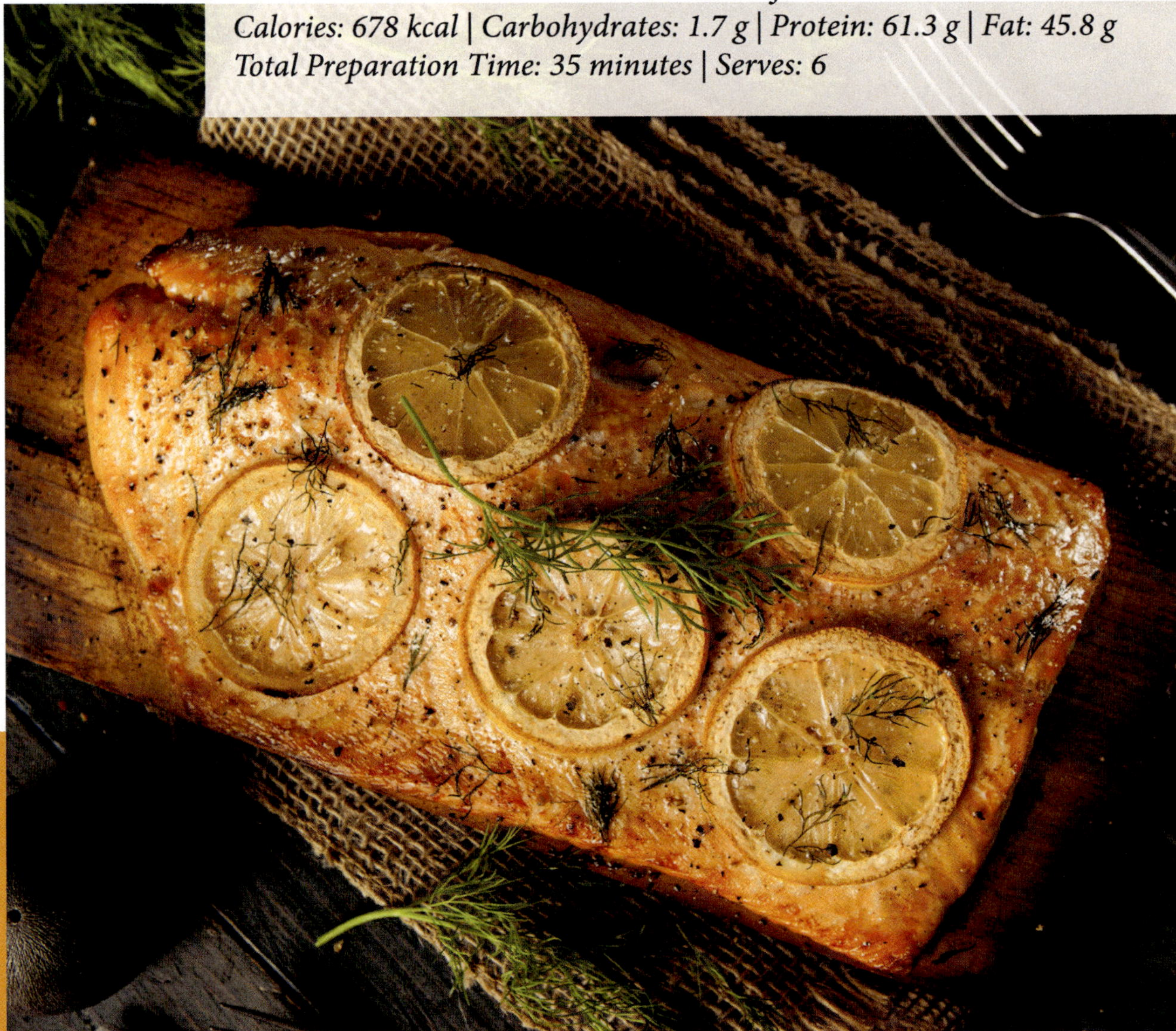

# INGREDIENTS

- *⅓ cup of vegetable oil*
- *1½ tbsp. of rice vinegar*
- *1 tsp. of sesame oil*
- *⅓ cup of soy sauce*
- *12 in. untreated cedar planks*
- *1 tbsp. of grated fresh ginger root*
- *1 tsp. of minced garlic*
- *2 lb. salmon fillets, skin removed*
- *¼ cup of chopped green onions*

# DIRECTIONS

1. Soak the cedar boards in warm water for at least 1 hour. (If you have time, soak longer.)
2. In a shallow dish, combine the vegetable oil, rice vinegar, sesame oil, soy sauce, green onions, ginger, and garlic.
3. Place the salmon fillets in the marinade mixture to coat well.
4. Cover and marinate in the refrigerator for 15 minutes to 1 hour.
5. Preheat the outside grill to a moderate heat setting.
6. Arrange the planks on top of the grate.
7. When the boards begin to smoke and crackle slightly, they are ready.
8. Arrange the salmon fillets on the planks, cover, and cook for approximately 20 minutes.
9. When you can split the fish with a fork, it is done. (After you remove it from the grill, it will continue to cook.)
10. Serve and enjoy!

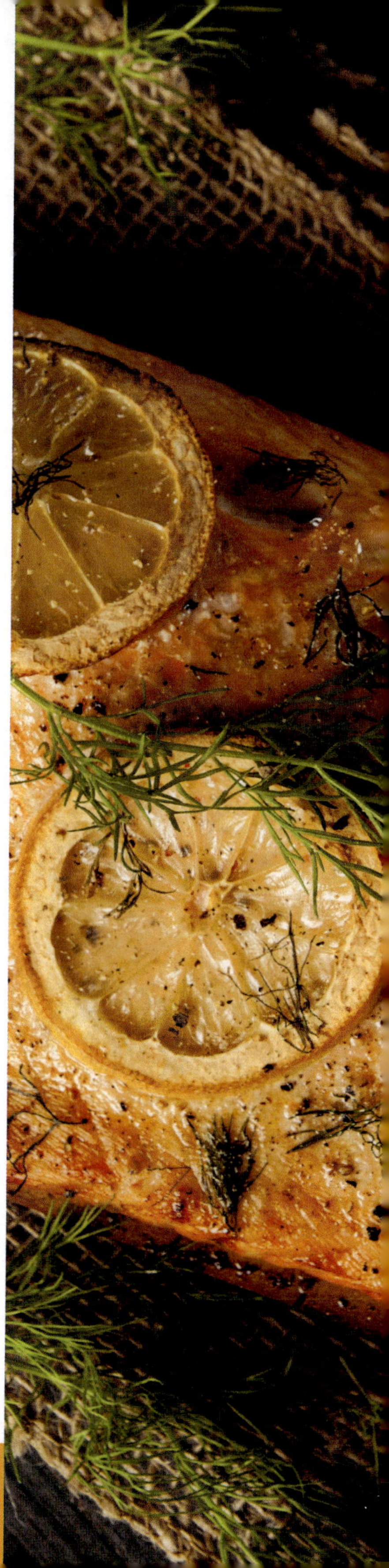

# *Marinated Tuna Steak*

***Nutritional Info:***

*Calories: 200 kcal | Carbohydrates: 3.7 g | Protein: 27.4 g | Fat: 7.9 g*
*Total Preparation Time: 51 minutes | Serves: 4*

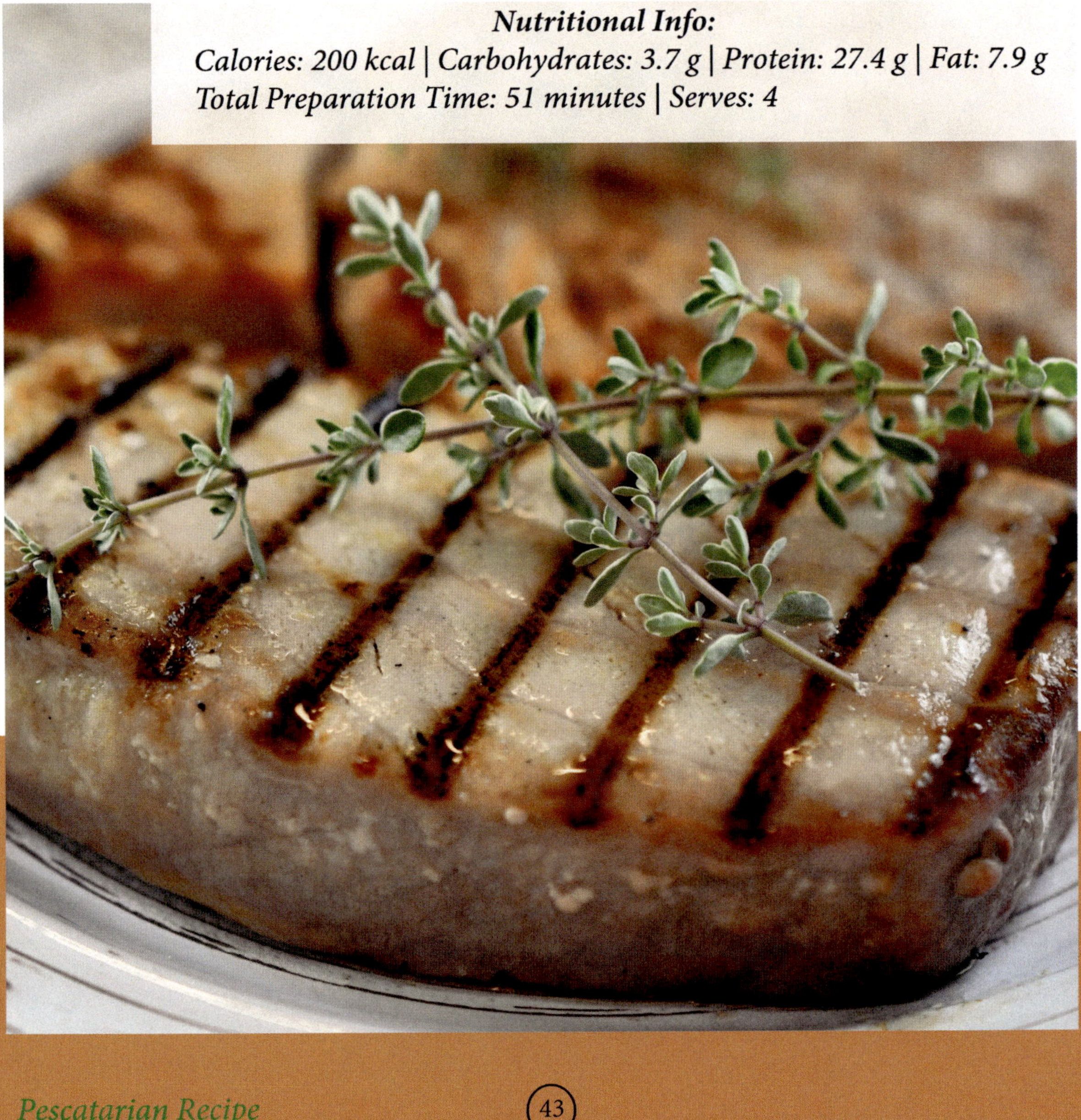

# INGREDIENTS

- *¼ cup of fresh orange juice*
- *2 tbsp. of olive oil*
- *1 tbsp. of lemon juice*
- *1 clove of garlic, minced*
- *¼ cup of soy sauce*
- *½ tsp. of fresh oregano, chopped*
- *½ tsp. of ground black pepper*
- *4 oz. tuna steaks*
- *2 tbsp. of fresh parsley, chopped*

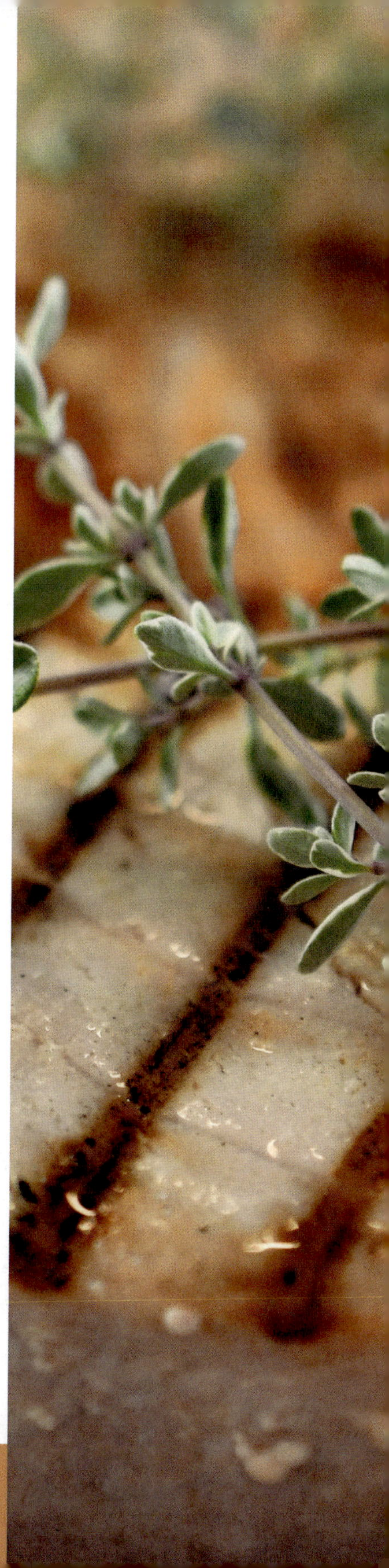

# DIRECTIONS

1. Combine the orange juice, soy sauce, olive oil, lemon juice, parsley, garlic, oregano, and pepper in a large non-reactive dish.
2. Turn the tuna steaks in the marinade to coat well.
3. Refrigerate covered and chill for at least 30 minutes.
4. Preheat grill to high and gently oil the grill grate.
5. Cook each side for about six minutes and then turn and baste with the marinade.
6. Cook for an additional 5 minutes, or until the desired degree of doneness is reached.
7. Serve and enjoy!

# *Vegetarian Baked Beans*

LOVE'S HOLISTIC NUTRITION

***Nutritional Info:***

*Calories: 214 kcal | Carbohydrates: 42.1 g | Protein: 10.6 g | Fat: 1 g*
*Total Preparation Time: 15 hrs, 10 minutes | Serves: 10*

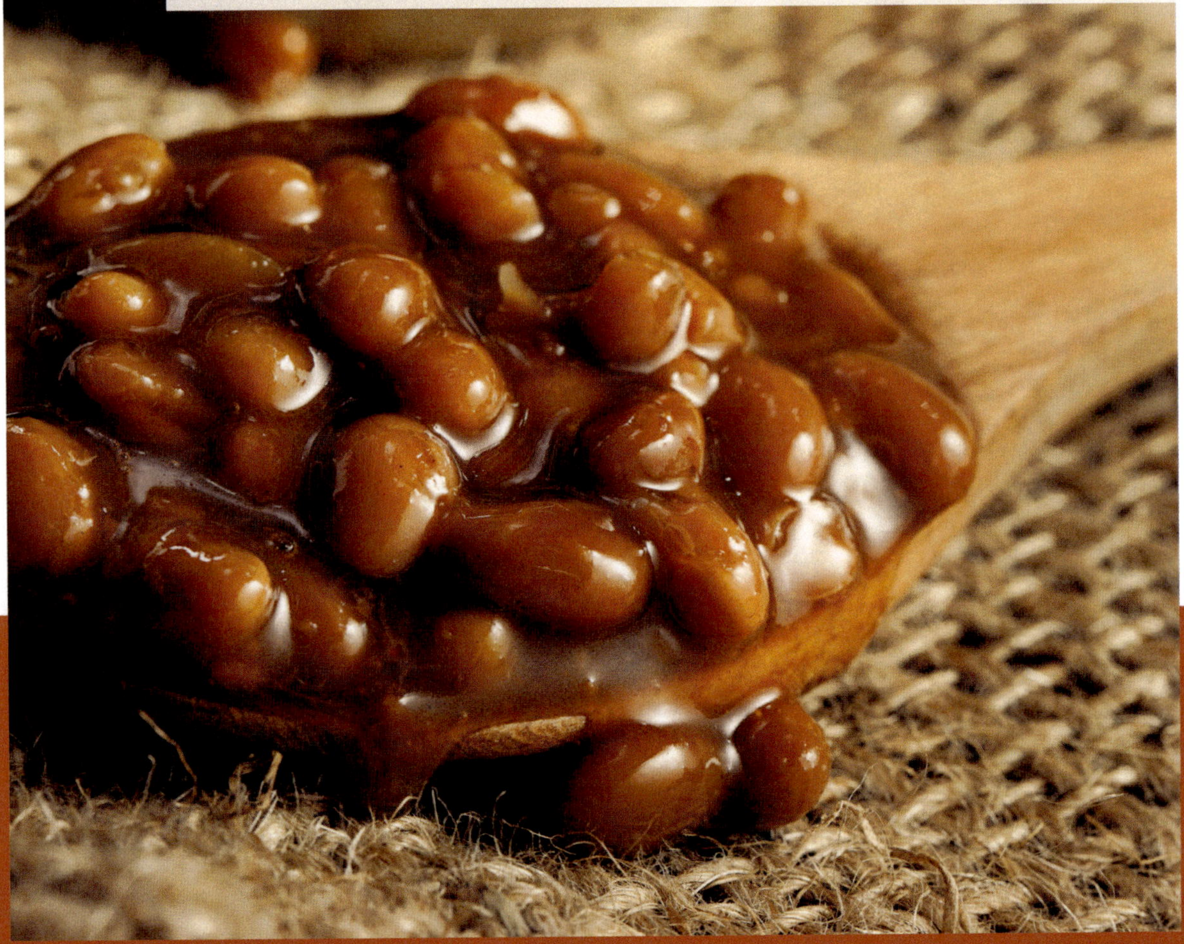

# INGREDIENTS

- *¼ cup of firmly packed brown sugar*
- *16 oz. package of dried navy beans*
- *2 cups of chopped sweet red onions*
- *2 tbsp. of apple cider vinegar*
- *2 tsp. of dry mustard*
- *1 clove garlic, chopped*
- *¼ tsp. of ground nutmeg*
- *Water, as needed*
- *¼ tsp. of ground cinnamon*
- *¼ tsp. of ground black pepper*
- *¼ cup of molasses*

# DIRECTIONS

1. Halfway fill a large container with navy beans and cover with several inches of water.
2. Set aside for 8 hours (overnight).
3. Drain the navy beans and place in a pot with 5 cups of water.
4. Bring the water to a boil.
5. Decrease the heat to a low level and continue cooking for approximately 1 hour.
6. Preheat the oven to 250°F (120°C).
7. In a 2-quart casserole dish with a lid, combine the beans, onion, brown sugar, molasses, vinegar, mustard, garlic, nutmeg, cinnamon, and pepper.
8. Cover the dish and bake for 5 to 7 hours in a preheated oven, stirring halfway through (adding water if it becomes too thick).
9. Remove the lid and continue baking for approximately 1 hour or more or until mixture has reduced to your desired thickness.
10. Serve and enjoy!

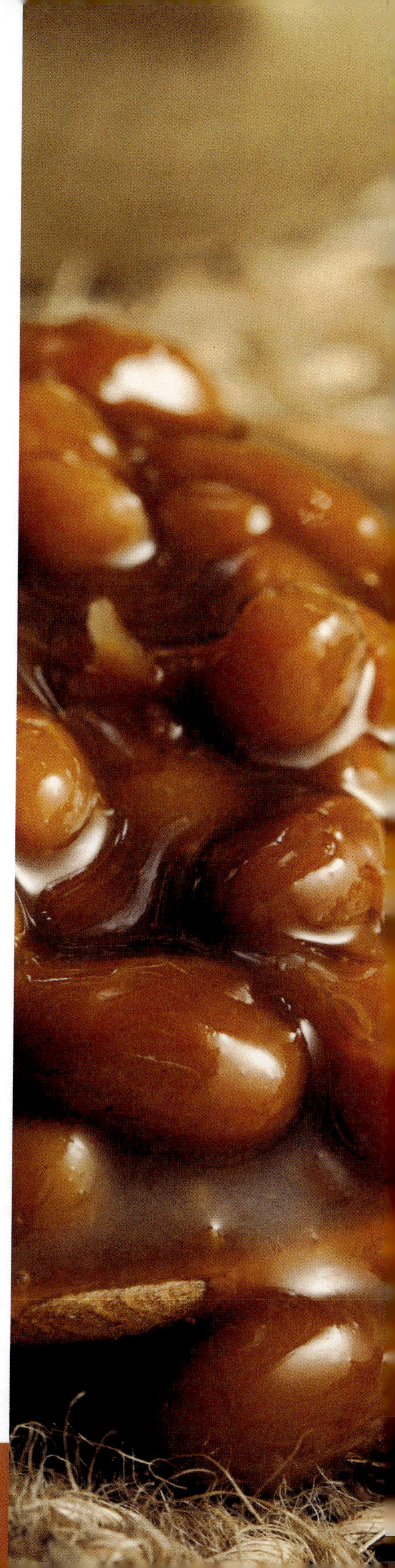

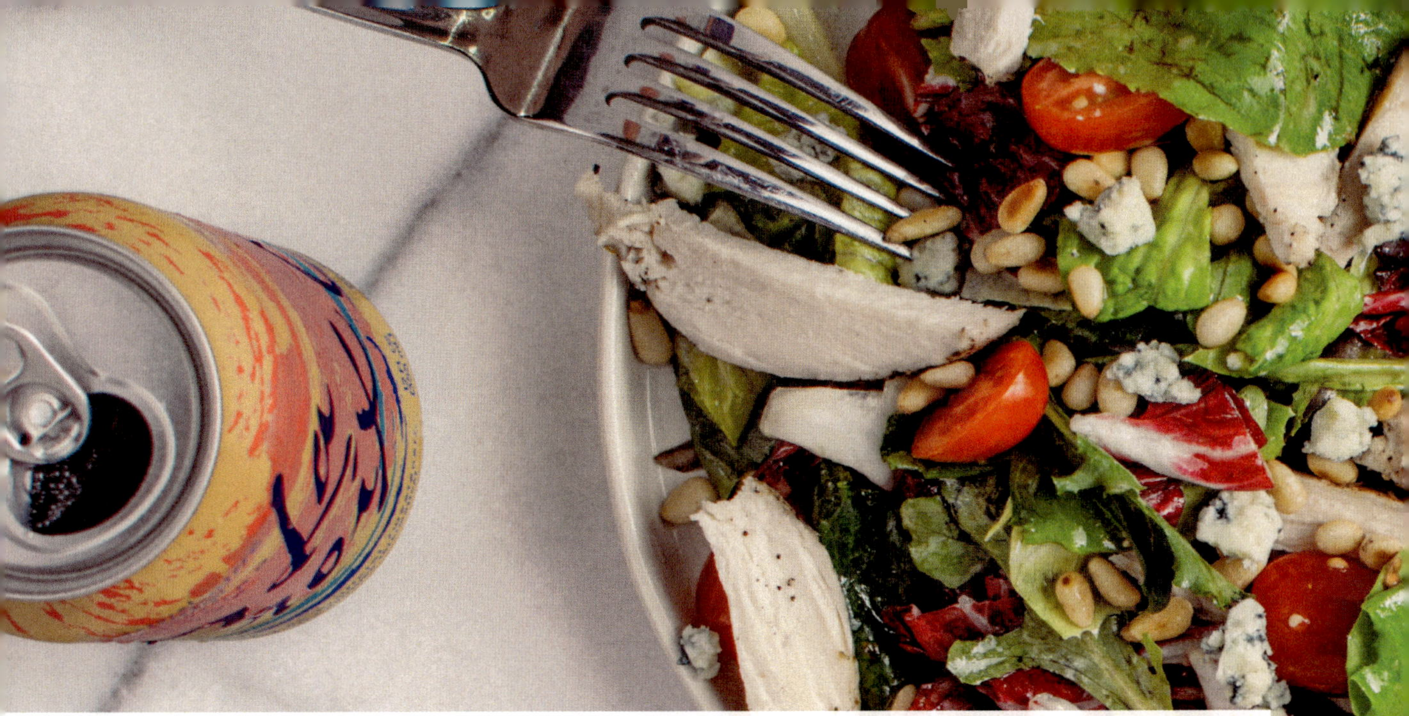

# *Dinner Recipes*

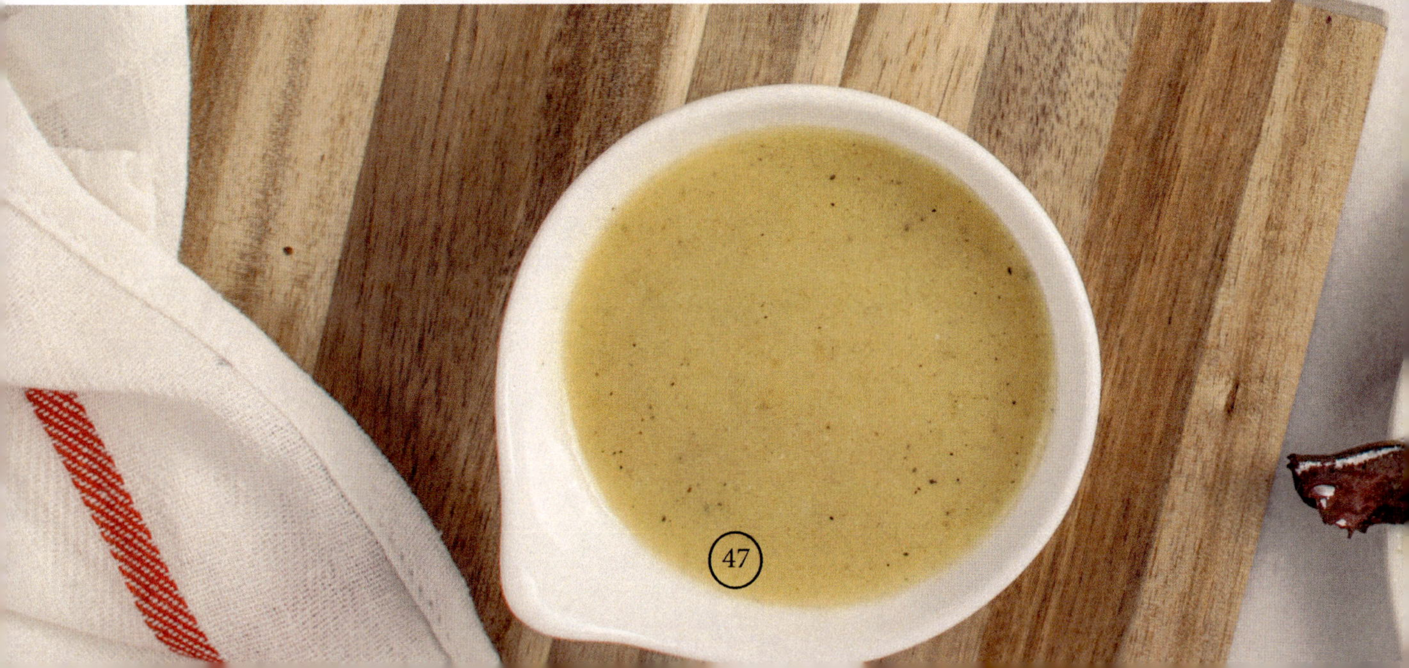

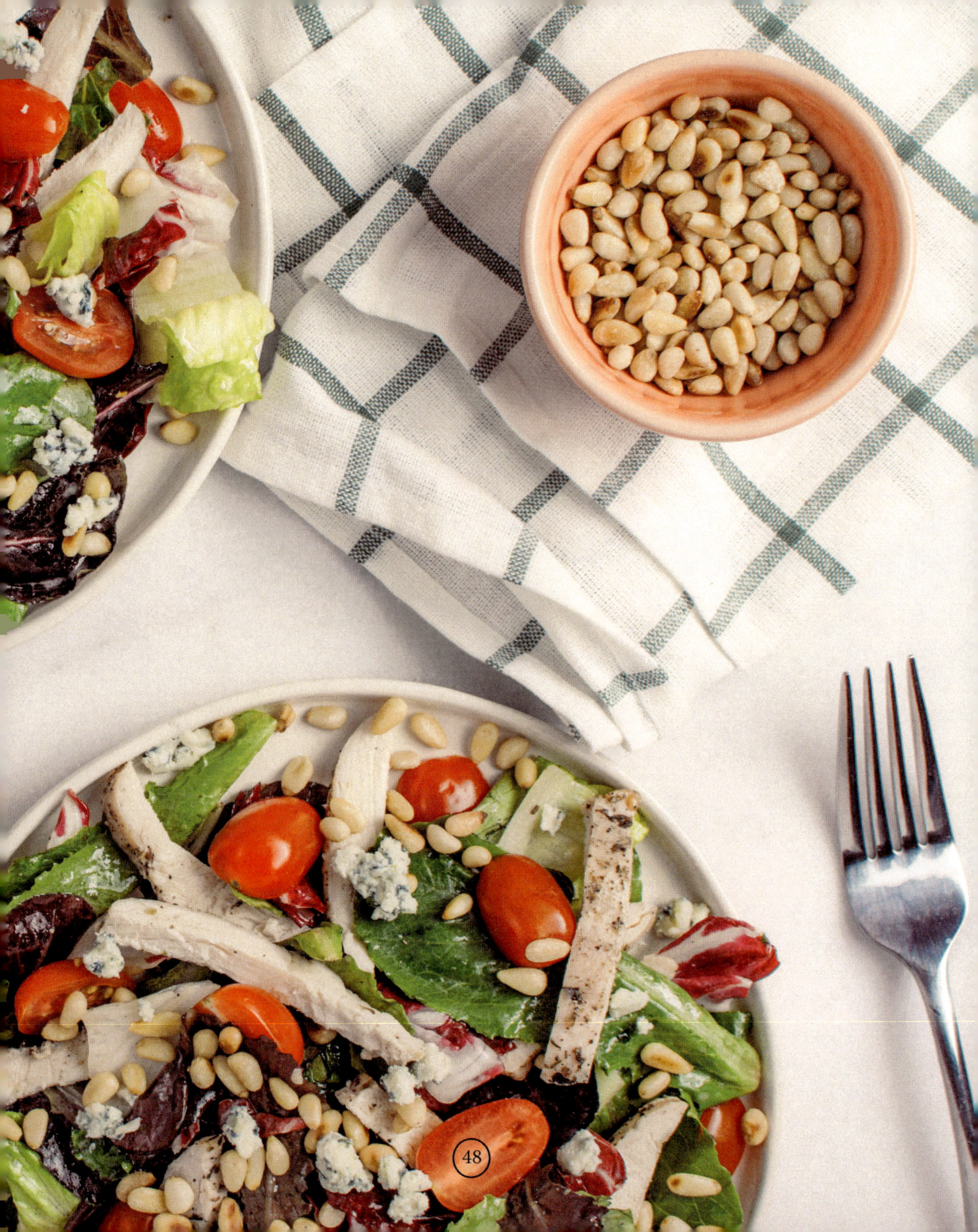

# Crispy Tofu with Black Pepper Sauce

**Nutritional Info:**

*Calories: 317 kcal | Carbohydrates: 20 g | Protein: 8 g | Fat: 23 g*
*Total Preparation Time: 40 minutes | Serves: 4*

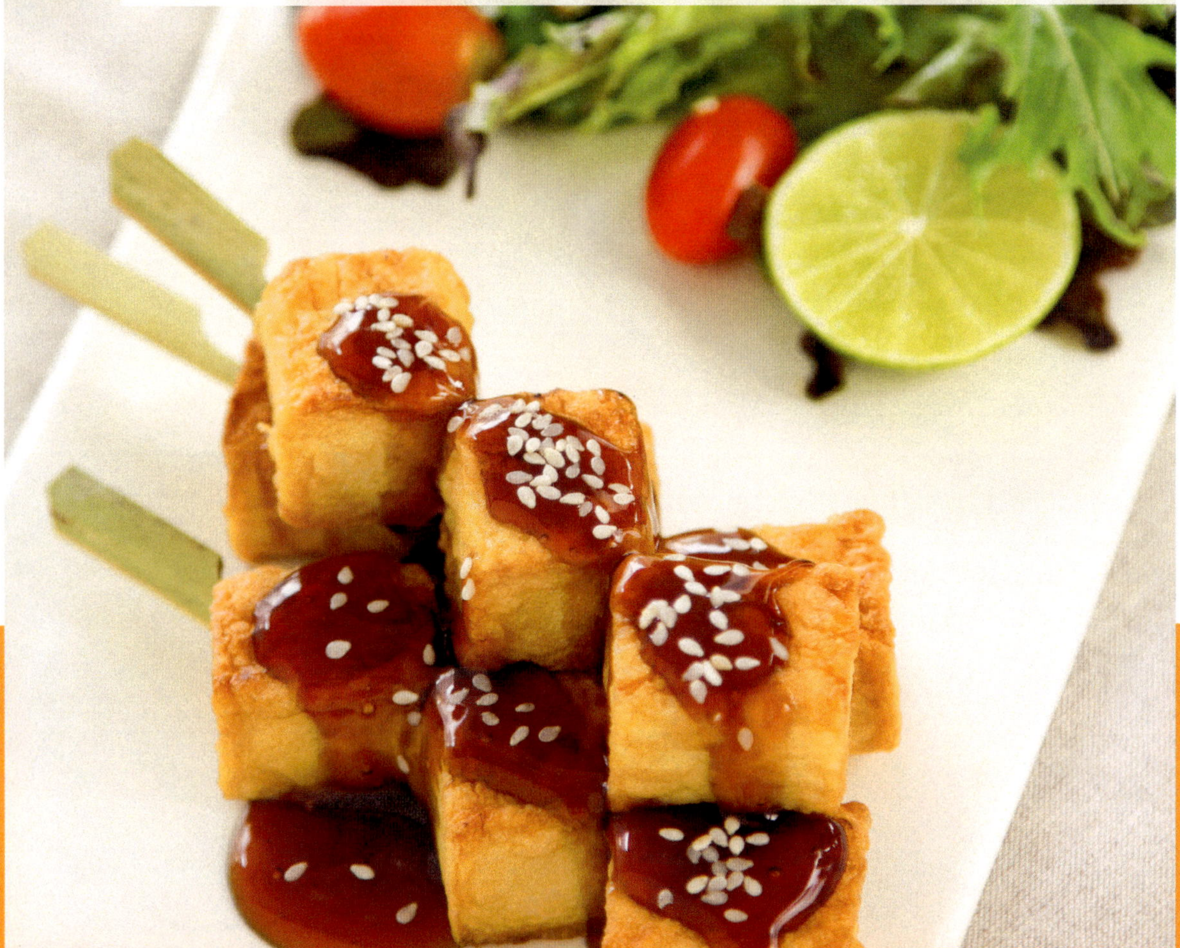

# INGREDIENTS

- *8 oz. of extra-firm tofu, drained*
- *3 tbsp. of cornstarch*
- *2 tbsp. of reduced sodium soy sauce*
- *2 tbsp. of chili garlic sauce*
- *1 tbsp. of brown sugar*
- *3 cloves of garlic, minced*
- *2 tsp. of grated ginger root*
- *1 tbsp. of rice vinegar*
- *4 green onions*
- *6 tbsp. of canola oil, divided*
- *8 oz. of fresh sugar snaps peas, trimmed and sliced*
- *1 tsp. of ground pepper*

# DIRECTIONS

1. Mix the cornstarch, soy sauce, garlic sauce, and brown sugar.
2. Mince the green onion whites; lightly slice the green bits.
3. Cut the tofu into ½ inch cubes and blot dry.
4. Toss the tofu in the cornstarch mixture.
5. Place the skillet over medium-high heat and warm 4 tbsp. of oil.
6. Cook, stirring continuously, until the tofu is golden brown and crisp (about 5-7 minutes).
7. Remove the tofu from the pan and pat dry with paper towels.
8. In a vast skillet, warm 1 tbsp. of oil in the same pan.
9. Stirfry the peas for 2-3 minutes, or until crisp and tender.
10. Then, remove the peas from the pan.
11. Heat the remaining oil in the same pan over medium-high heat. Cook for 30 seconds before adding pepper.
12. Stirfry the garlic, ginger, and minced green onions for 30 to 45 seconds.
13. Add the soy sauce mixture and simmer, constantly stirring, until slightly thickened.
14. Take off the heat and mix in the tofu and peas.
15. Garnish with thinly sliced green onions.
16. Serve and enjoy!

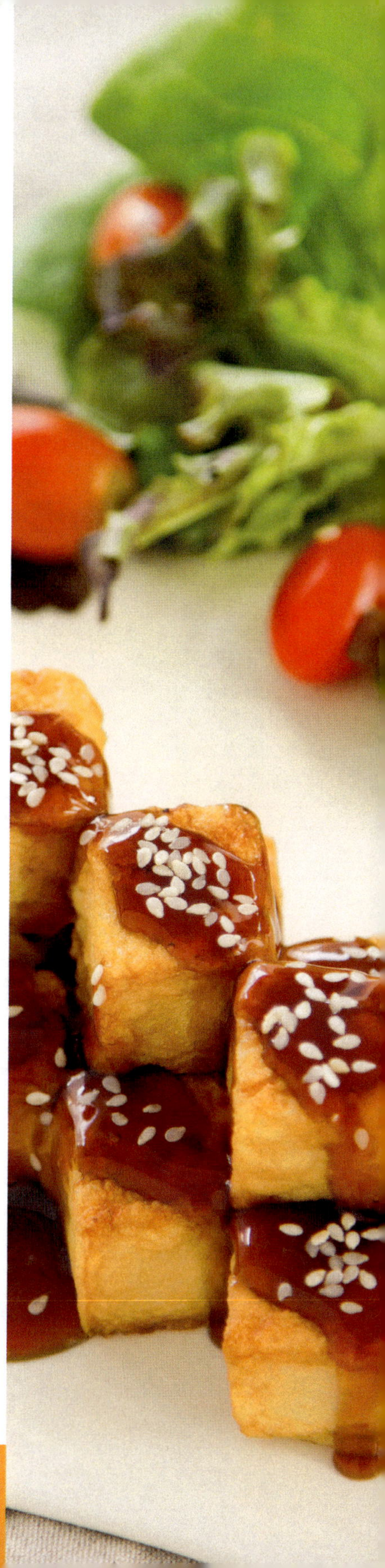

# *Gnocchi with Pesto Sauce*

***Nutritional Info:***

*Calories: 328 kcal | Carbohydrates: 53 g | Protein: 10 g | Fat: 8 g*

*Total Preparation Time: 32 minutes | Serves: 4*

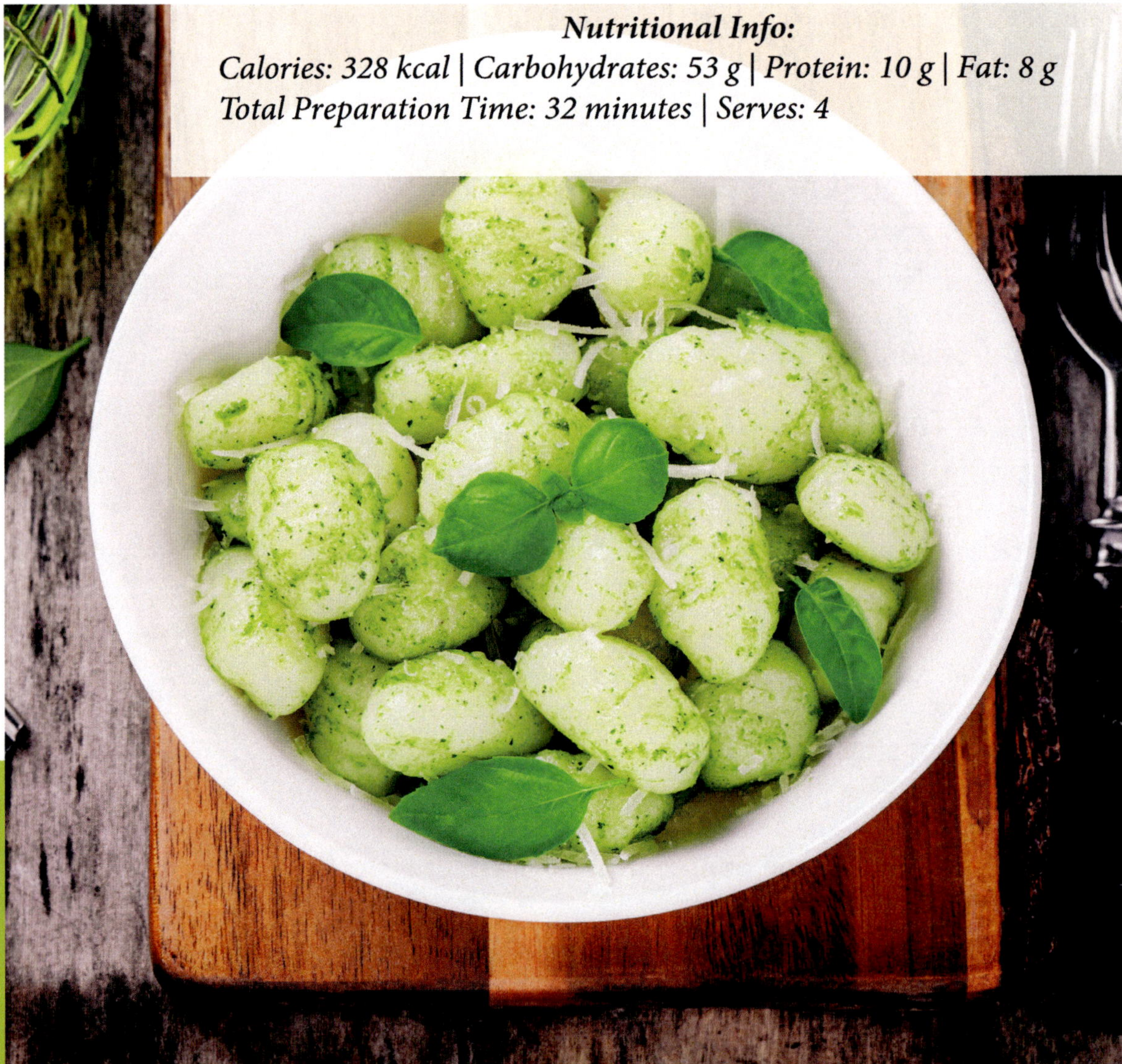

# *INGREDIENTS*

- *2 tsp. of olive oil*
- *16 oz. of potato gnocchi*
- *1 cup of tomatoes, chopped*
- *Pine nuts, toasted*
- *1 cup of diced zucchini*
- *½ cup of sweet yellow pepper, chopped*
- *¼ cup of prepared pesto*

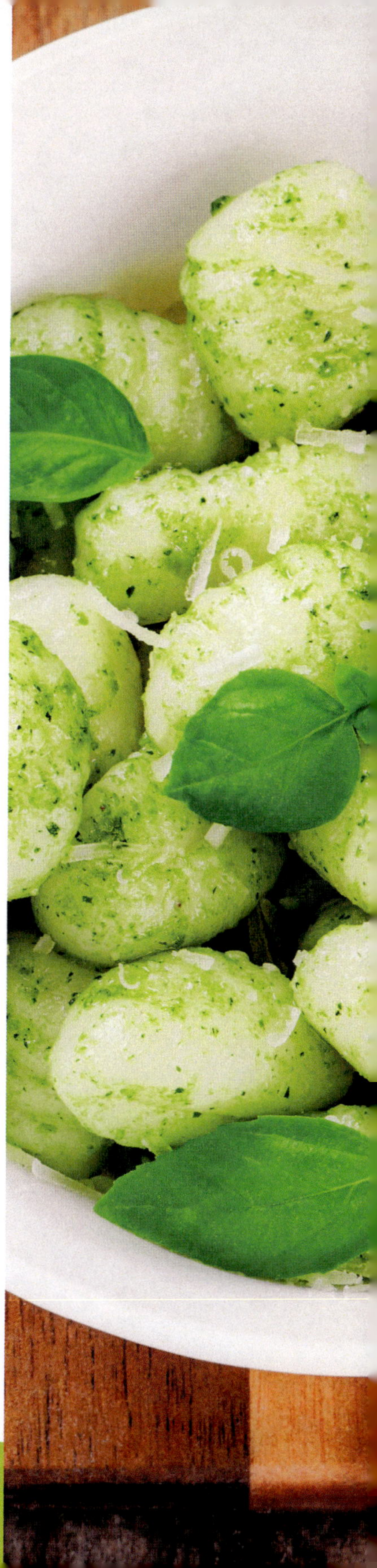

# *DIRECTIONS*

1. Cook the gnocchi according to the package directions.
2. Drain the gnocchi.
3. Heat the olive oil over medium-high heat.
4. Sauté the zucchini and pepper until tender.
5. Add the pesto and gnocchi, stirring gently to coat.
6. Stir in the tomatoes.
7. If desired, top with pine nuts.
8. Serve and enjoy!

# Mushroom Bean Bourguignon

**Nutritional Info:**

*Calories: 235 kcal | Carbohydrates: 34 g | Protein: 10 g | Fat: 6g*
*Total Preparation Time: 1 hour, 40 minutes | Serves: 10*

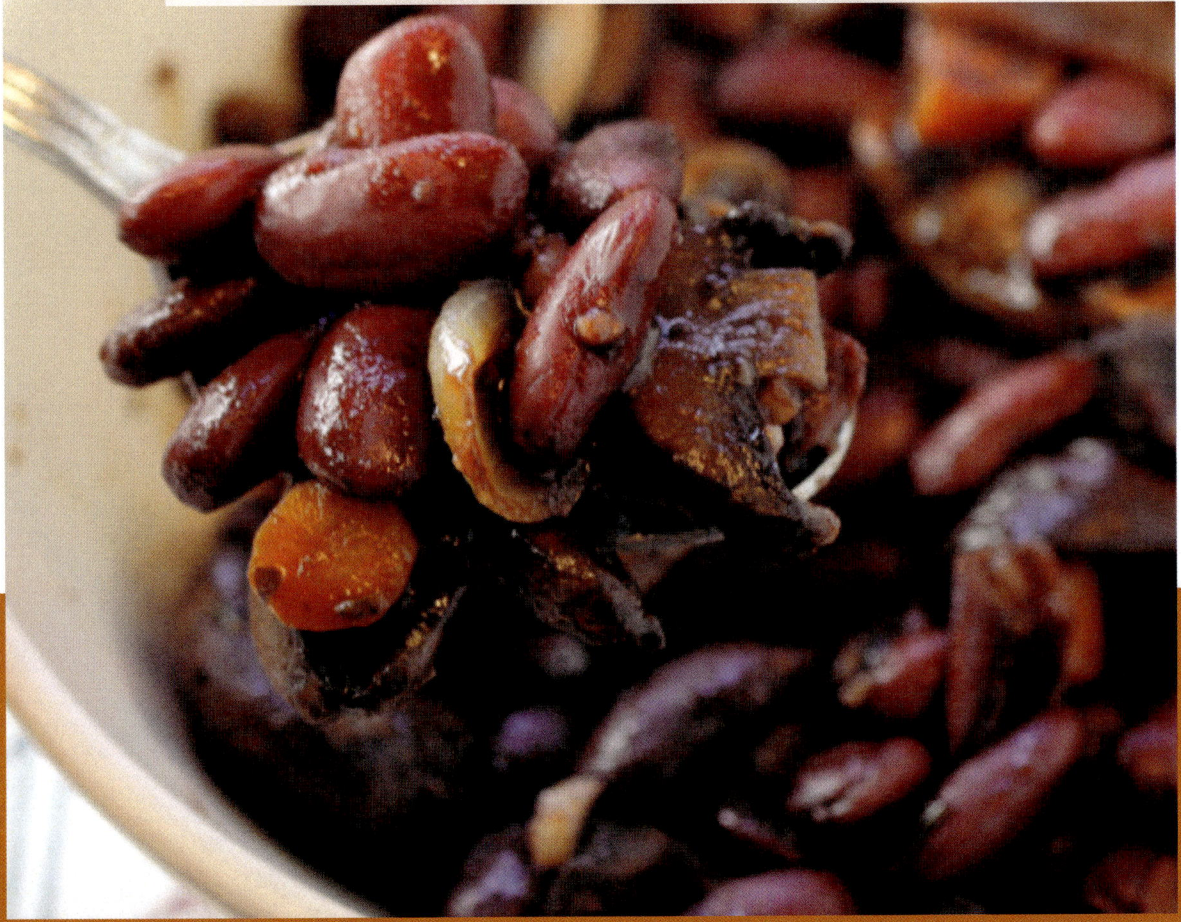

# INGREDIENTS

- *4 tbsp. of olive oil, divided*
- *5 carrots, cut into pieces*
- *14½ oz. of frozen pearl onions*
- *3 tbsp. of all-purpose flour*
- *2 onions, halved and sliced*
- *2 cloves of garlic, minced*
- *3¼ dry red wine*
- *2 cups of mushroom broth, divided*
- *1 tsp. of salt*
- *8 Portobello mushrooms, cut in pieces*
- *1 tbsp. of tomato paste*
- *1 tsp. of minced fresh thyme*
- *½ tsp. of pepper*
- *3 oz. of navy beans, rinsed and drained*

# DIRECTIONS

1. Heat 2 tbsp of oil over medium-high heat in a Dutch oven.
2. Add the carrots and onions; cook until soft.
3. Add the garlic and cook for an additional 1 minute.
4. Remove the carrots, pearl onions, and garlic from the pan.
5. In the same pan, heat 1 tbsp. of oil on medium-high heat.
6. Add half of the mushrooms and cook until gently brown.
7. Remove from the pan and repeat with 1 tbsp. of oil and the remaining mushrooms.
8. Reintroduce all of the mushrooms to the pan.
9. Add the tomato paste and simmer, constantly stirring for 1 minute.
10. Bring to a boil with the wine, 1½ cups of broth, salt, thyme, pepper, and carrot combination.
11. Decrease the temperature to low and cook covered for 25 minutes.
12. Add the pearl onions, garlic, and beans; cook for another 30 minutes.
13. Whisk the flour and remaining liquid in a small bowl until smooth; stir into pan.
14. Bring to a boil; cook and whisk for about 2 minutes, or until slightly thickened.
15. Serve and enjoy!

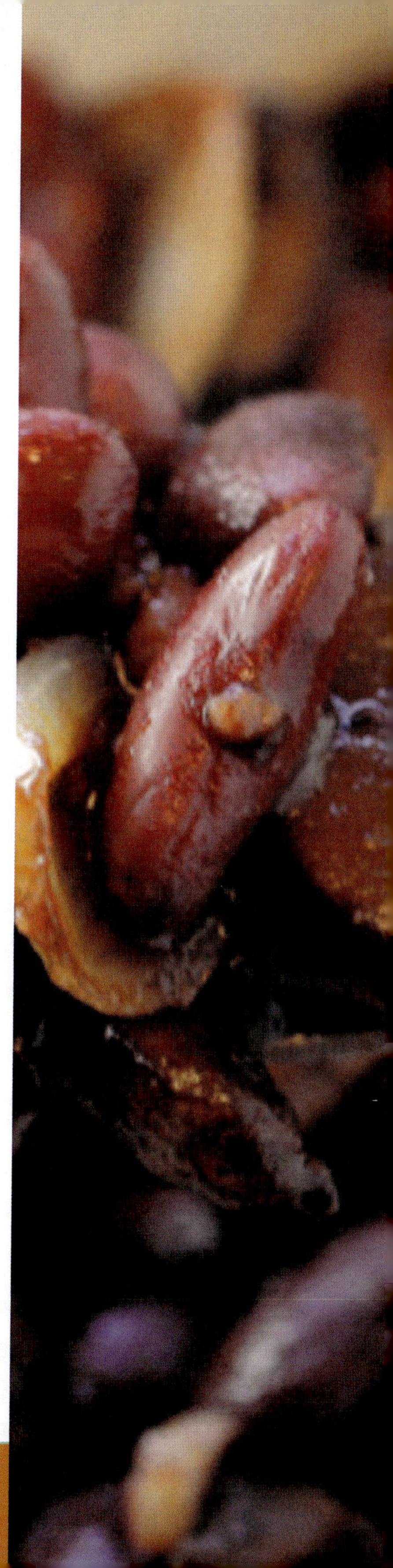

# *Pan-Seared Salmon*

***Nutritional Info:***

*Calories: 371 kcal | Carbohydrates: 1.7 g | Protein: 33.7 g | Fat: 25.1 g*
*Total Preparation Time: 20 minutes | Serves: 4*

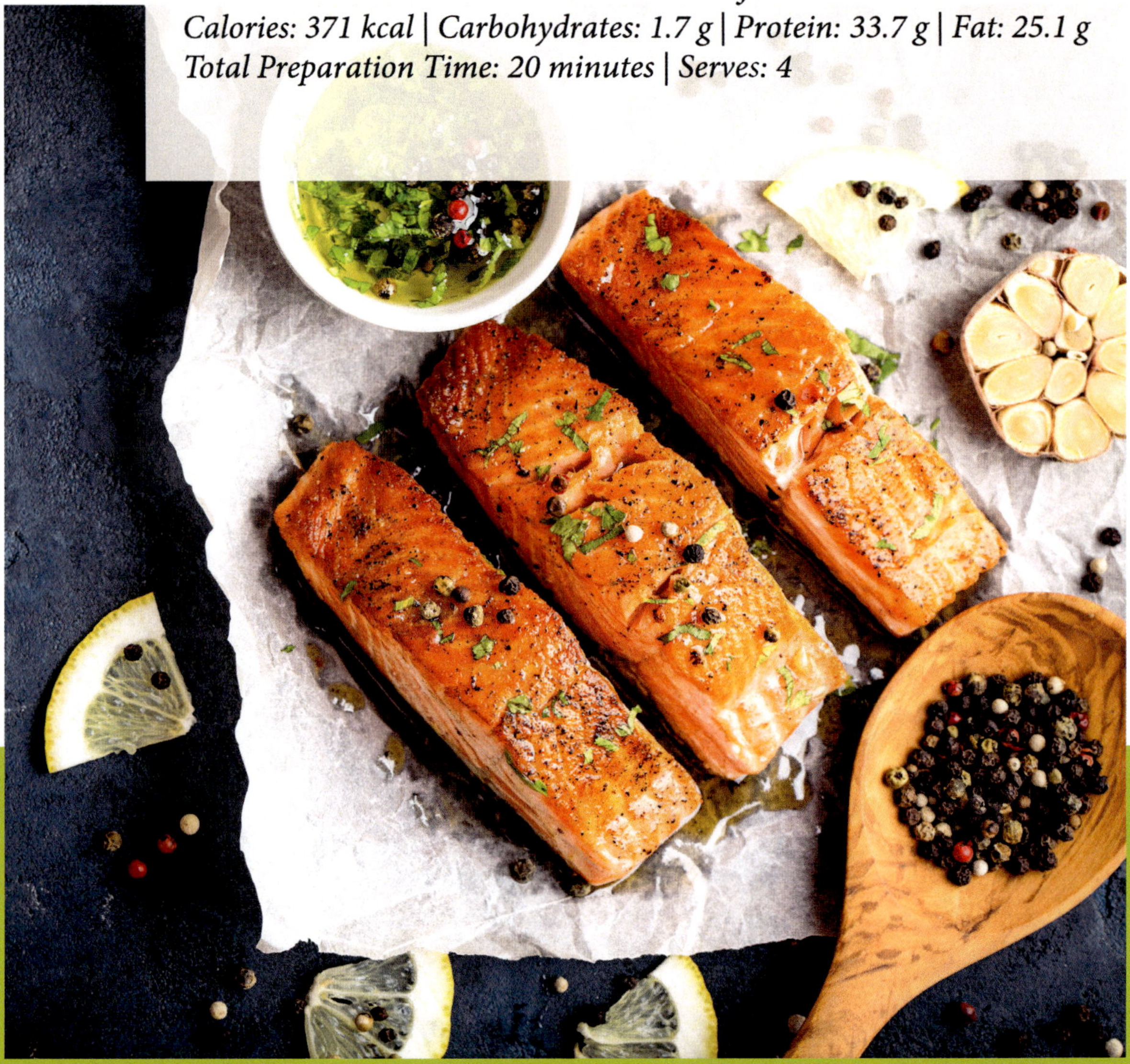

# *INGREDIENTS*

- *2 tbsp. of olive oil*
- *Pinch of salt*
- *Pinch of ground black pepper*
- *2 tbsp. of capers*
- *6 oz. of salmon fillets*
- *4 lemon slices*

# *DIRECTIONS*

1. Preheat a large, heavy skillet over medium heat.
2. Arrange the salmon on a plate and drizzle with olive oil.
3. Increase the heat to high and add the salmon to the skillet.
4. Cook for 3 minutes.
5. Season the salmon with capers, salt, and pepper, to taste.
6. Cook for another 5 minutes, or until the salmon is browned and easily flakes with a fork.
7. Individually plate the salmon and garnish with lemon slices.
8. Serve and enjoy!

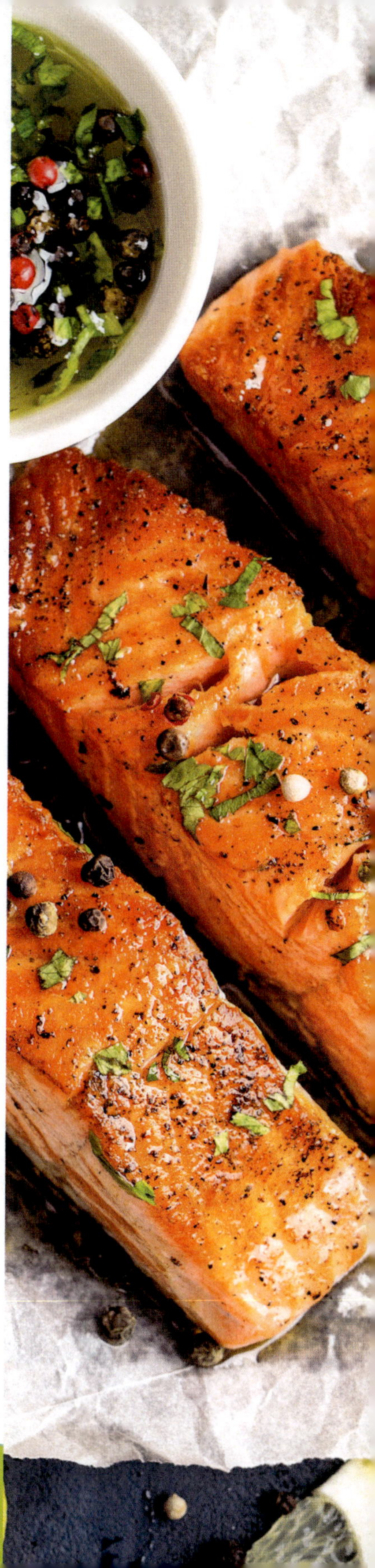

# *Sun-Dried Tomato Linguine*

LOVE'S HOLISTIC NUTRITION

**Nutritional Info:**

*Calories: 542 kcal | Carbohydrates: 68 g | Protein: 23 g | Fat: 21 g*

*Total Preparation Time: 25 minutes | Serves: 6*

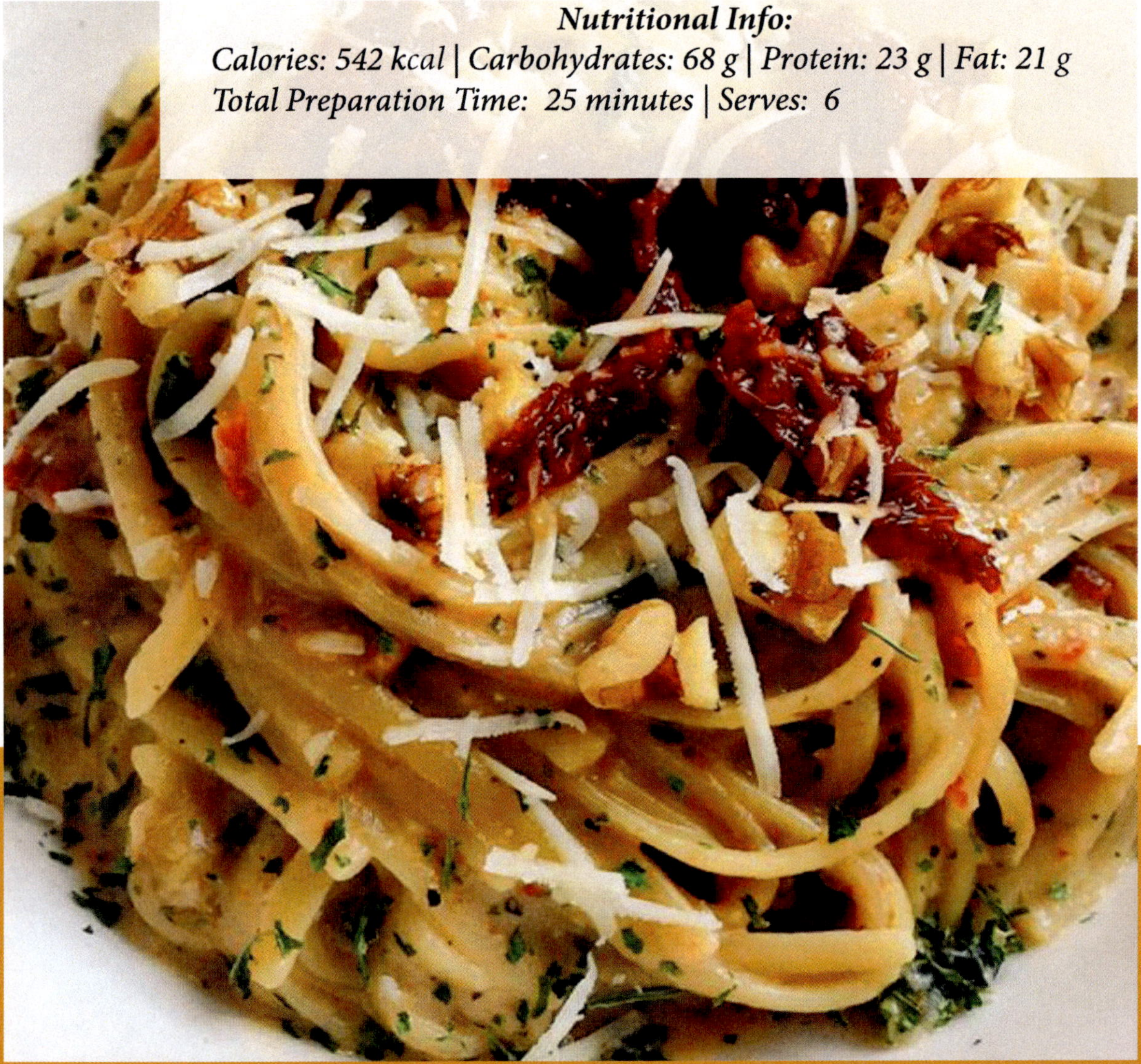

# *INGREDIENTS*

- *16 oz. of linguine*
- *½ cups of crumbled feta cheese*
- *7 oz. of julienned tomatoes, oil-packed and sun-dried*
- *6 garlic cloves, grated*
- *1 tbsp. of lemon juice*
- *½ cup of fresh parsley, minced*
- *1½ cups of parmesan cheese, shredded*

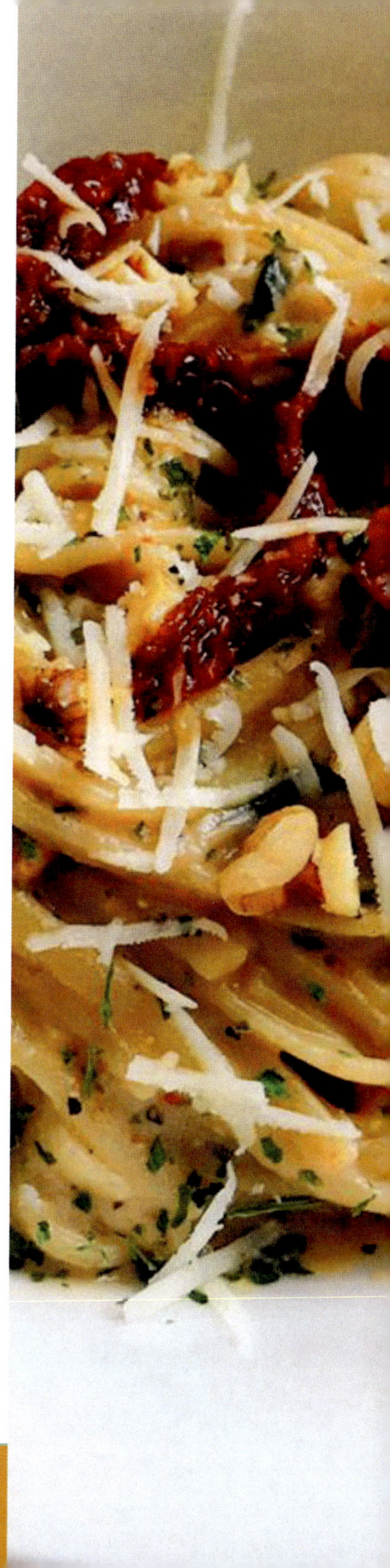

# *DIRECTIONS*

1. Prepare the linguine al dente, based on the instructions given on the package in a 6 qt. stockpot.
2. Drain the linguine, reserving ½ cup pasta water on the side.
3. Return the linguine to the pot (without water in it).
4. Drain the tomatoes, reserving 2 tbsp. of oil.
5. Microwave the garlic and reserved oil for 45 seconds on high in a small microwave-safe bowl.
6. Combine the drained tomatoes and lemon juice.
7. Toss the linguine with tomato sauce.
8. Add in the parsley, cheeses, and just enough of the reserved pasta water to keep the mixture moist.
9. Serve and enjoy!

# Garden Vegetable Gnocchi

**Nutritional Info:**
Calories: 402 kcal | Carbohydrates: 57 g | Protein: 13 g | Fat: 14 g
Total Preparation Time: 35 minutes | Serves: 4

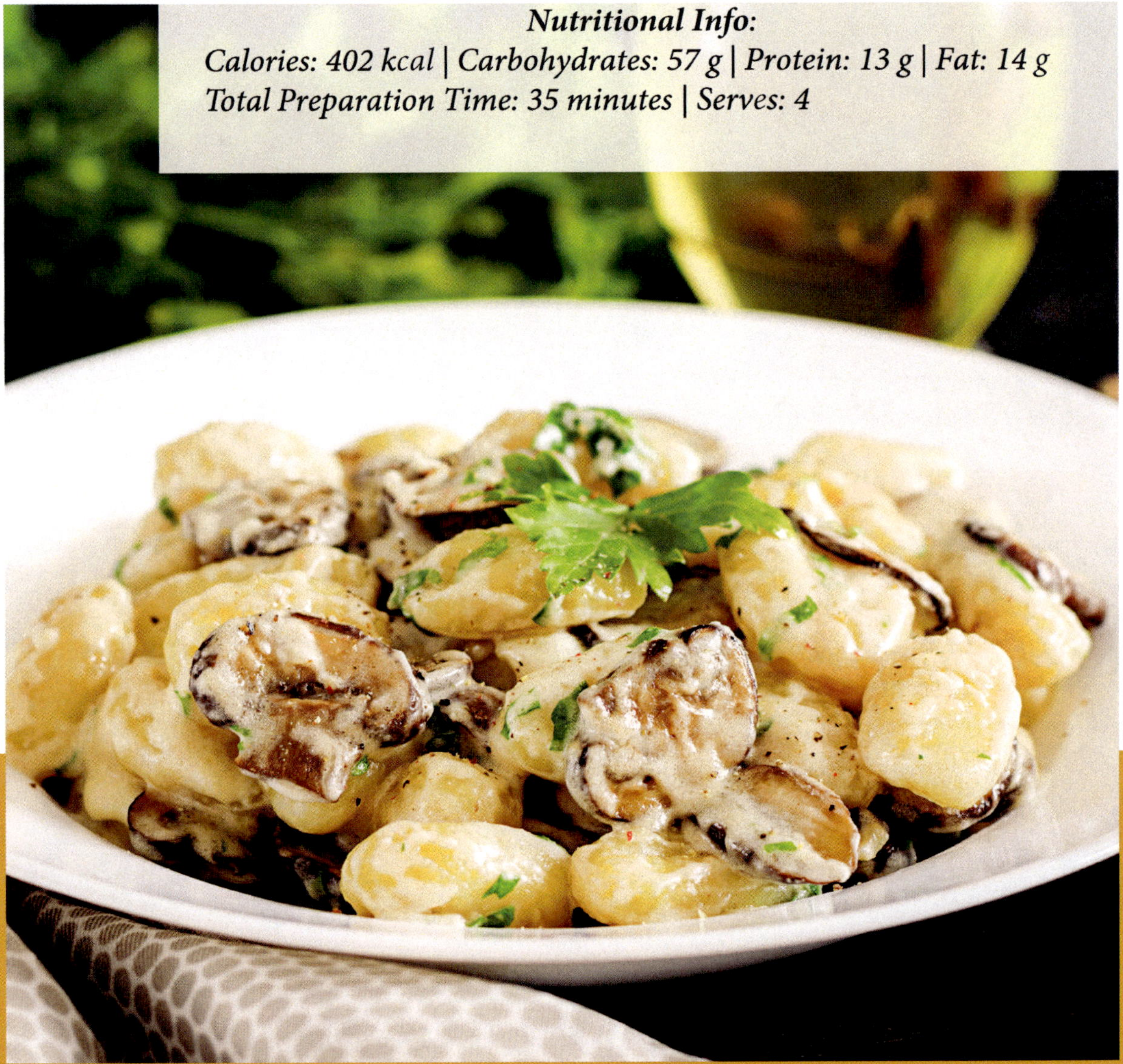

# *INGREDIENTS*

- *1 medium sweet red pepper, sliced*
- *8 oz. of fresh mushrooms, chopped*
- *1 tbsp. of olive oil*
- *¼ tsp. of salt*
- *2 small yellow summer squash, sliced*
- *¼ tsp. of pepper*
- *½ cup of Alfredo sauce*
- *¼ cup of pre-ready pesto*
- *16 oz. of potato gnocchi*
- *Fresh basil, chopped (optional)*

# *DIRECTIONS*

1. Preheat the oven to 400°F.
2. In a greased baking dish, toss the vegetables with oil, salt, and pepper.
3. Roast for 18-22 minutes, stirring once, or until tender.
4. Meanwhile, boil the gnocchi according to the package directions in a large pot.
5. Drain and reintroduce to the pan.
6. Combine the roasted vegetables, Alfredo sauce, and pesto in a large mixing bowl.
7. Sprinkle with basil, if desired.
8. Serve and enjoy!

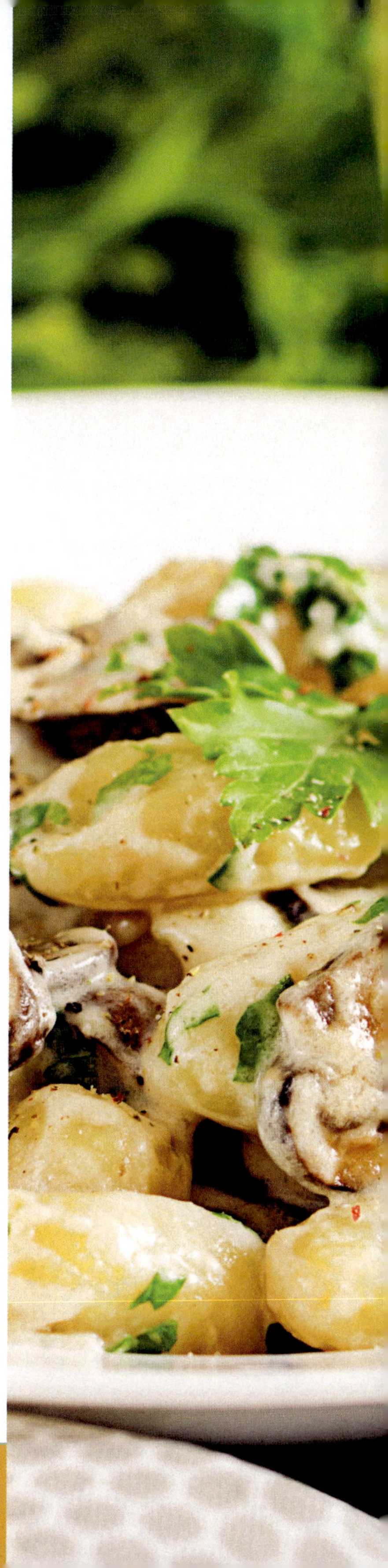

# Mushroom and Brown Rice Hash with Poached Eggs

**Nutritional Info:**

*Calories: 282 kcal | Carbohydrates: 26 g | Protein: 13 g | Fat: 13g*
*Total Preparation Time: 30 minutes | Serves: 4*

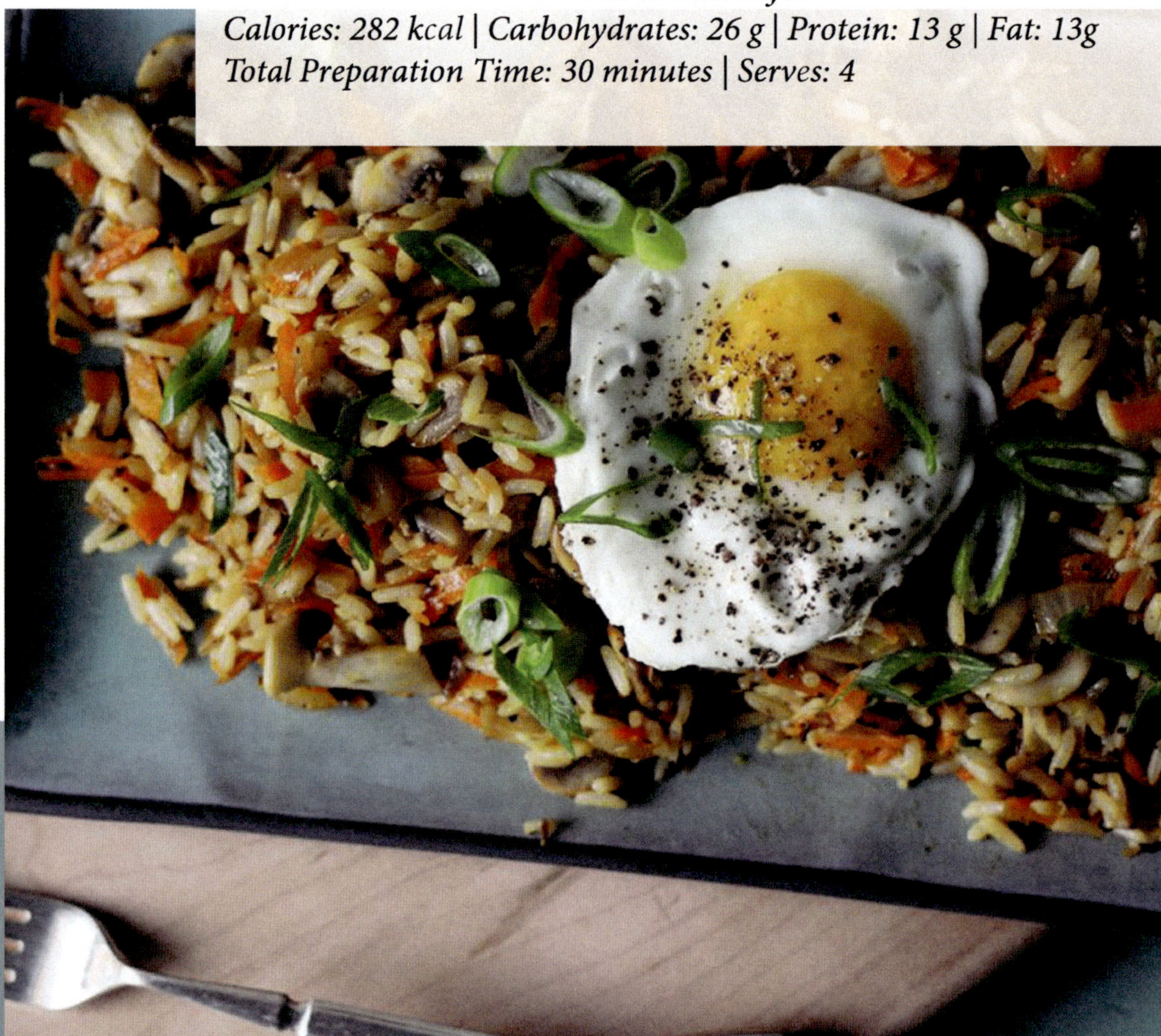

# INGREDIENTS

- *2 tbsp. of olive or canola oil*
- *1 lb. of baby Portobello mushrooms, sliced*
- *½ cup of sweet onion, chopped*
- *8.75 oz. of pre-cooked brown rice*
- *1 large carrot, sliced*
- *½ tsp. of salt*
- *2 green onions, slices*
- *¼ tsp. of pepper*
- *¼ tsp. of caraway seeds*
- *4 large eggs*

# DIRECTIONS

1. Place the skillet over medium-high heat.
2. Add the oil to the skillet and heat it.
3. Add the mushrooms and sauté it for 5-7 minutes, or until lightly browned.
4. Add the sweet onion and cook for 1 minute.
5. Add the cooked rice and carrots; stir and cook for about 4-5 minutes.
6. Heat the green onions, salt, pepper, and caraway seeds.
7. Fill a large saucepan with 2-3 inches of water and bring to a boil.
8. Reduce to a low simmer.
9. Break the cold eggs into a small bowl, one at a time.
10. While holding the bowl close to the water's surface, pour the egg into the water.
11. Cook for 3-5 minutes in an uncovered pan, or until the egg whites are completely set and the yolks begin to thicken, but not quite firm.
12. Using a slotted spoon, separate the eggs from water and place on top of the rice mixture.
13. Serve and enjoy!

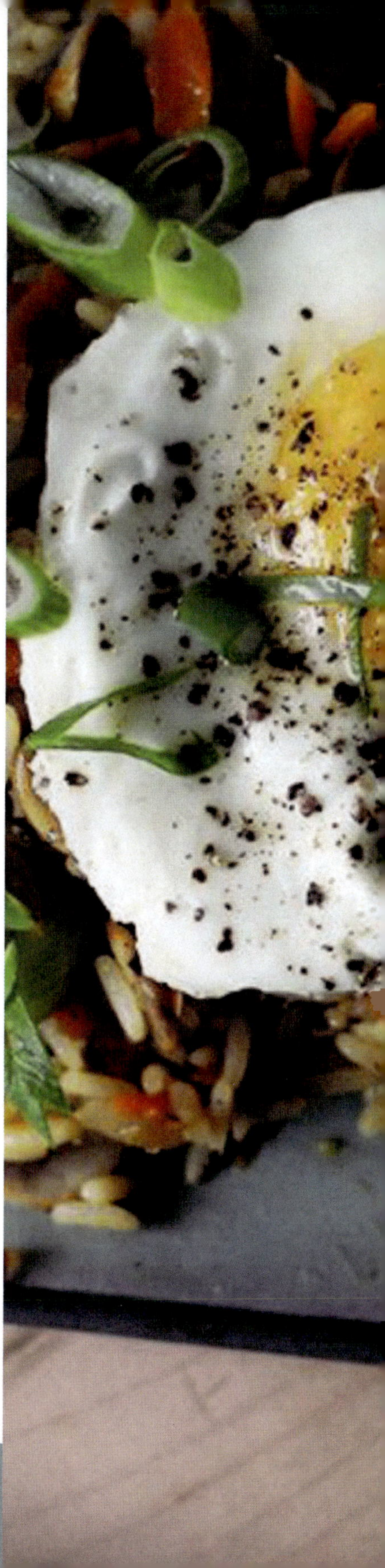

# One Pan Chicken and Veggies

**Nutritional Info:**

*Calories: 405kcal | Carbohydrates: 38 g |Protein: 43g | Fat: 9 g*

*Total Preparation Time: 30 minutes | Serves: 4*

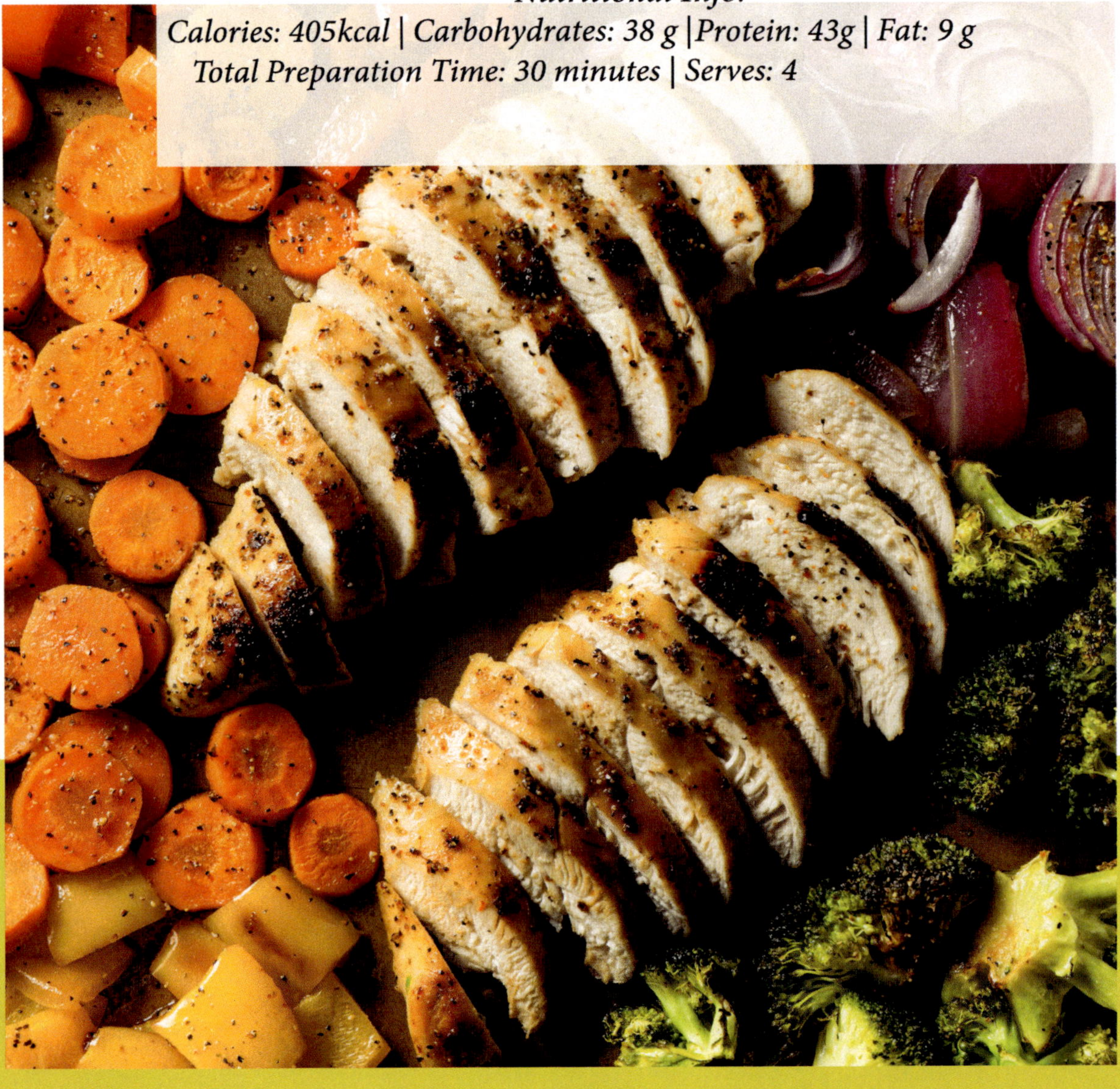

# *INGREDIENTS*

- *1 bunch of asparagus, trimmed and cut into small pieces*
- *1 cup of chicken stock*
- *1 tsp. of arrowroot starch*
- *3 cups of baby potatoes, quartered*
- *¼ cup of balsamic vinegar*
- *1 lb. of boneless skinless chicken breast, cut into 1 in. cubes*
- *½ zucchini, cut into bite-sized pieces*
- *¼ tsp of salt*
- *½ cup of feta cheese, crumbled (for serving)*
- *2 tsp of olive oil, divided*
- *¼ cup of pomegranate arils (for serving)*
- *Salt and pepper, to taste*

# *DIRECTIONS*

1. Heat 1 tbsp. of oil in the pan over medium heat.
2. Add potatoes, season with salt and pepper, and cover.
3. Cook for about 15 minutes, or until tender.
4. Add the zucchini and asparagus to the pan and stir.
5. Cover and cook for 5 minutes.
6. Move the potatoes, zucchini, and asparagus to a large bowl and sprinkle with arrowroot starch and toss.
7. Add the chicken to the pan with 1 tbsp. of olive oil and cook for 8-10 minutes.
8. Add the potatoes, zucchini, and asparagus back into the in the pan along with the chicken stock, salt, and balsamic vinegar.
9. Cook, while occasionally stirring for 3-5 minutes.
10. Sprinkle with feta cheese and pomegranates arils.
11. Serve and enjoy!

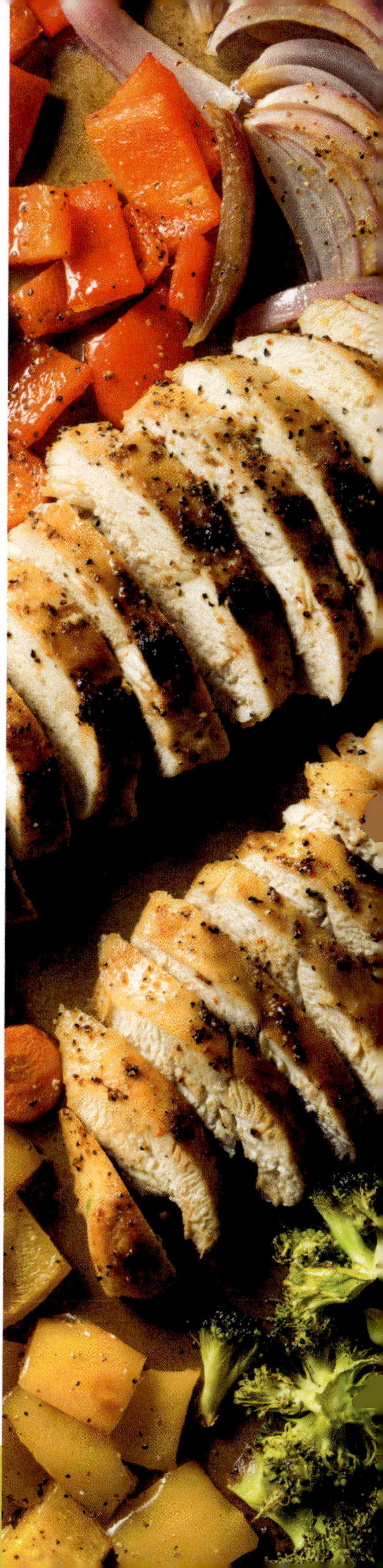

# Balsamic Glazed Beef Skewers

**Nutritional Info:**

*Calories: 485 k, Carbohydrates: 13 g | Protein: 26 g | Fat: 5 g*
*Total Preparation Time: 30 minutes | Serves: 4*

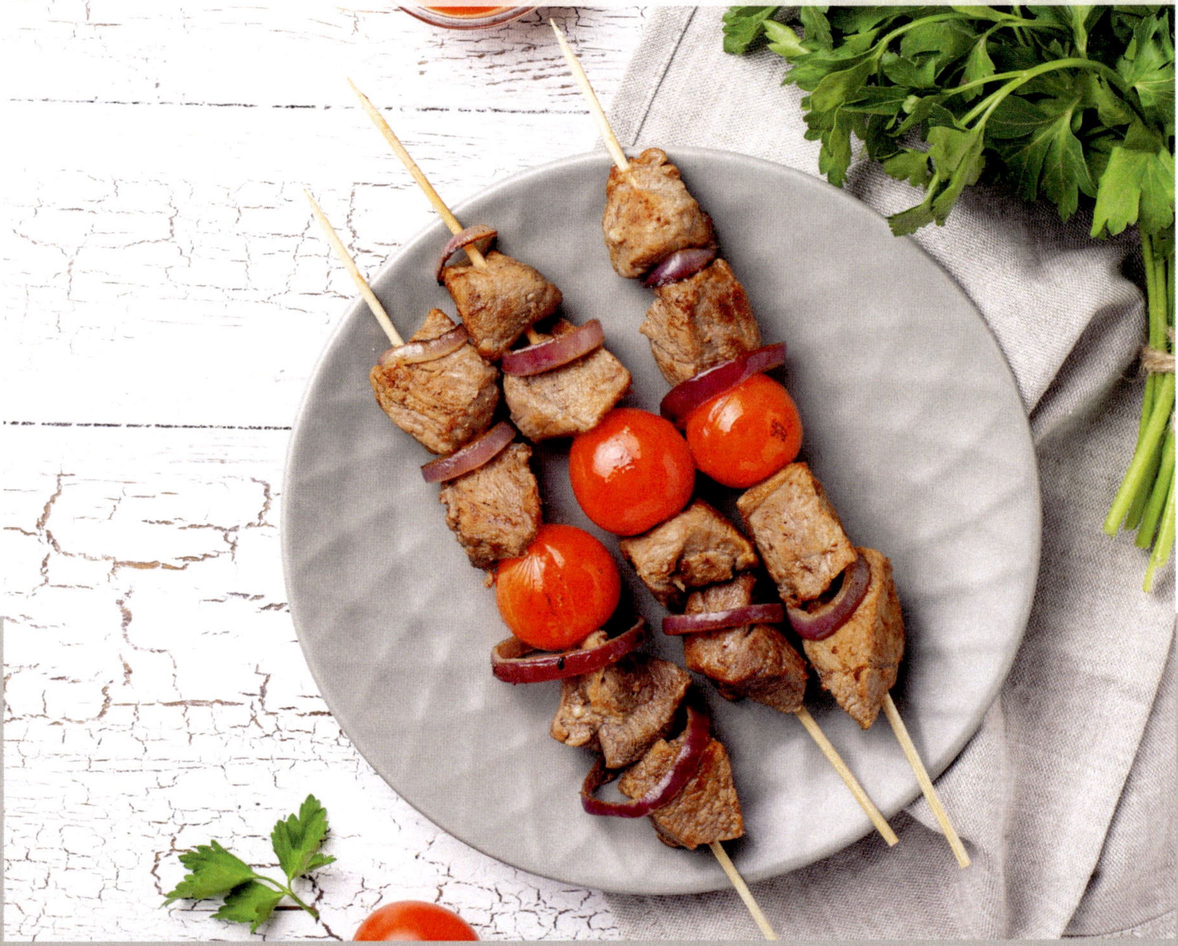

# *INGREDIENTS*

- *2 cups of cherry tomatoes*
- *¼ cup of balsamic vinaigrette*
- *1 tsp. of Dijon mustard*
- *1 pound of beef top sirloin steak, cut into 1 in. cubes*
- *¼ cup barbecue sauce*

# *DIRECTIONS*

1. In a large bowl, whisk the barbecue sauce, mustard, and vinaigrette until blended.
2. Set aside ¼ cup of the mixture for basting.
3. Add the beef to remaining mixture; toss to coat.
4. Thread the tomatoes and beef on 4 soaked wooden (or metal) skewers.
5. Lightly grease the grill rack.
6. Cover and grill the skewers over medium heat for 7-9 minutes, or until cooked as desired.
7. During the last 3 minutes, turn and baste frequently with the reserved mixture.
8. Serve and enjoy!

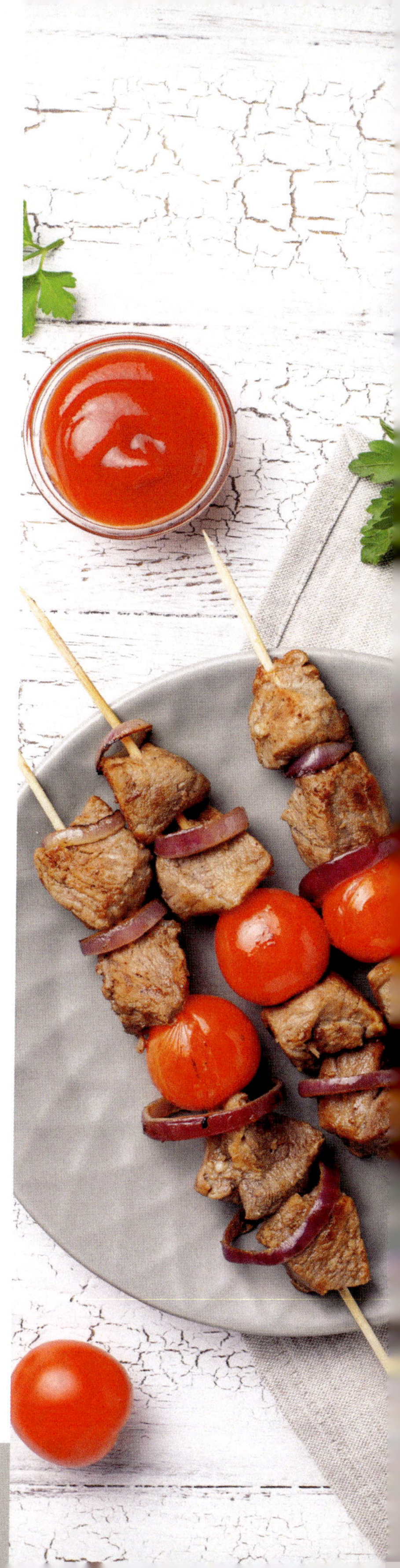

# *Vegan Black Bean Soup*

**Nutritional Info:**

*Calories: 361 kcal | Carbohydrates: 55 g | Protein: 24 g | Fat: 5 g*

*Total Preparation Time: 45 minutes | Serves: 6*

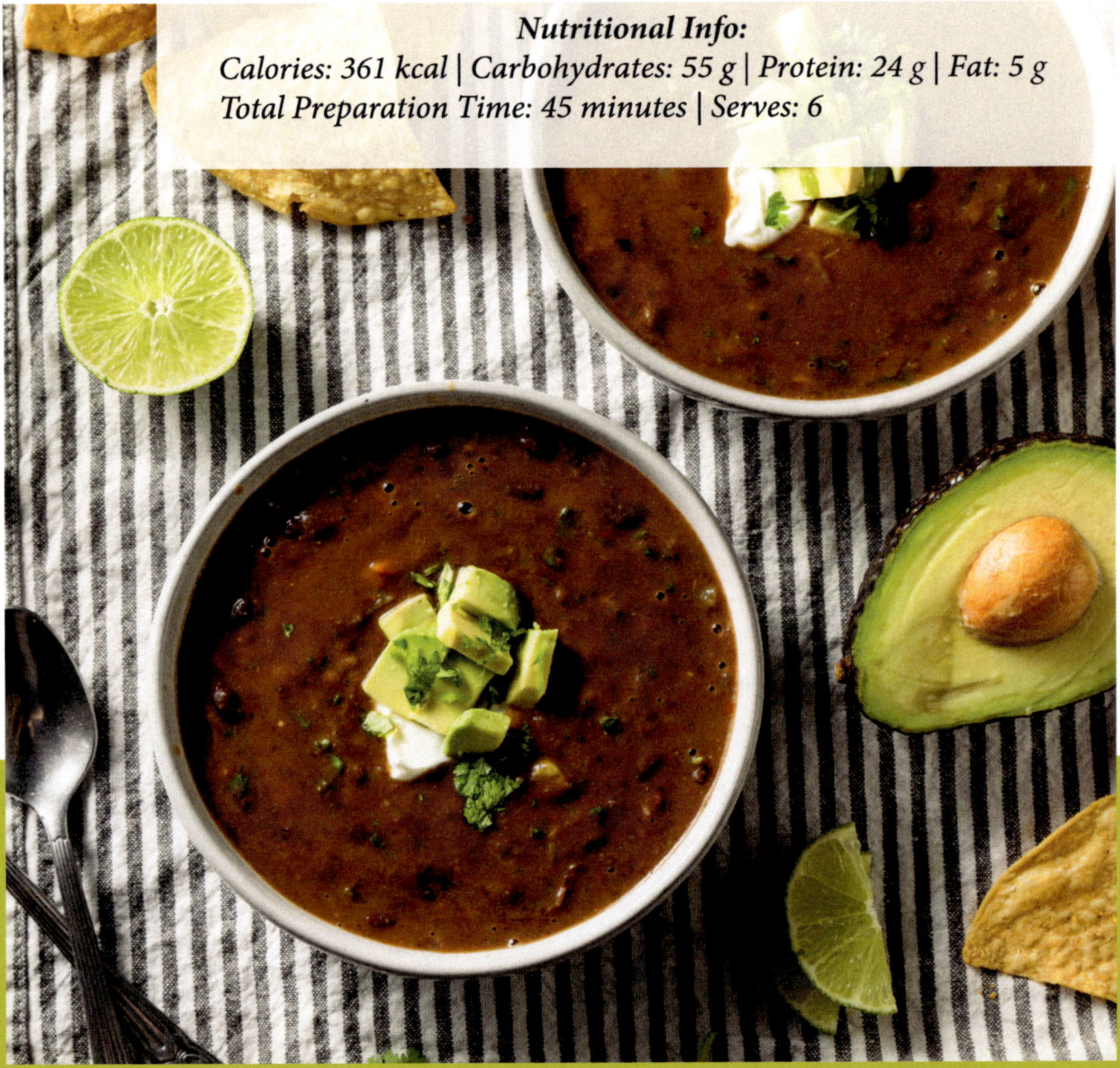

# *INGREDIENTS*

- *4 cups of vegetable broth*
- *1 tbsp. of olive oil*
- *1 large red onion, chopped*
- *1 stalk of celery, chopped*
- *2 carrots, chopped*
- *4 cloves of garlic, minced*
- *2 tbsp. of chili powder*
- *2 tsp. of ground cumin*
- *(4) 15 oz. cans of black beans*
- *15 oz. can of whole kernel corn*
- *14.5 oz. of tomatoes, chopped*
- *Pinch of black pepper*

# *DIRECTIONS*

1. Place the large saucepan over medium-high heat.
2. Add the oil and sauté the onion, celery, carrots, and garlic for 5 minutes.
3. Season with chili powder, cumin, and black pepper; cook for an additional 1 minute.
4. Combine the vegetable broth, 2 cans of beans, and corn in a large mixing bowl.
5. Add the mixture to the saucepan.
6. Increase the heat under the saucepan to high and bring it to a boil.
7. In a food processor, pulse the remaining 2 cans of beans and tomatoes until smooth.
8. Stir this into the boiling soup mixture.
9. Reduce to medium heat, and cook for 15 minutes.
10. Serve and enjoy!

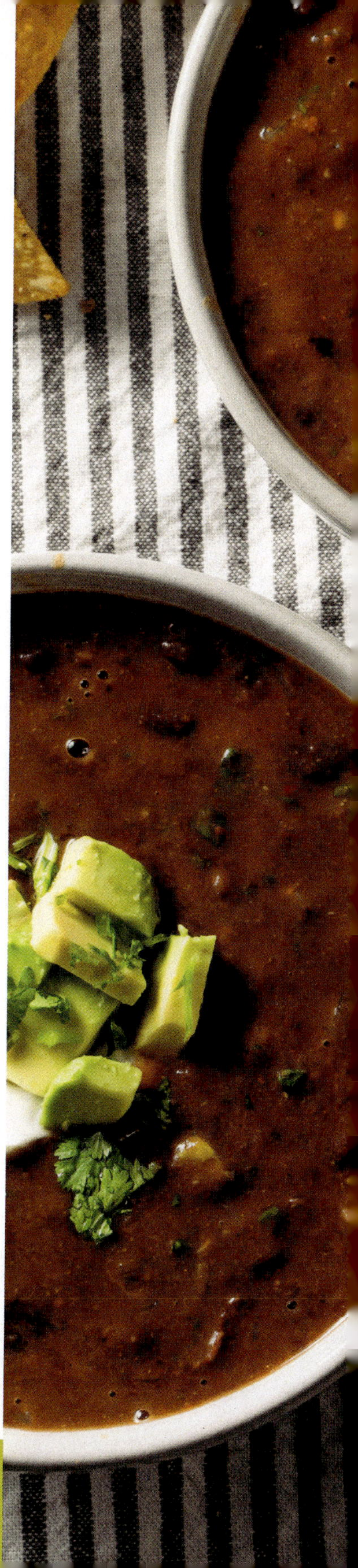

# White Beans with Artichoke and Tomato

**Nutritional Info:**

*Calories: 410 kcal | Carbohydrates: 24 g, Protein: 10 g, Fat: 8 g*

*Total Preparation Time: 25minutes | Serves: 4*

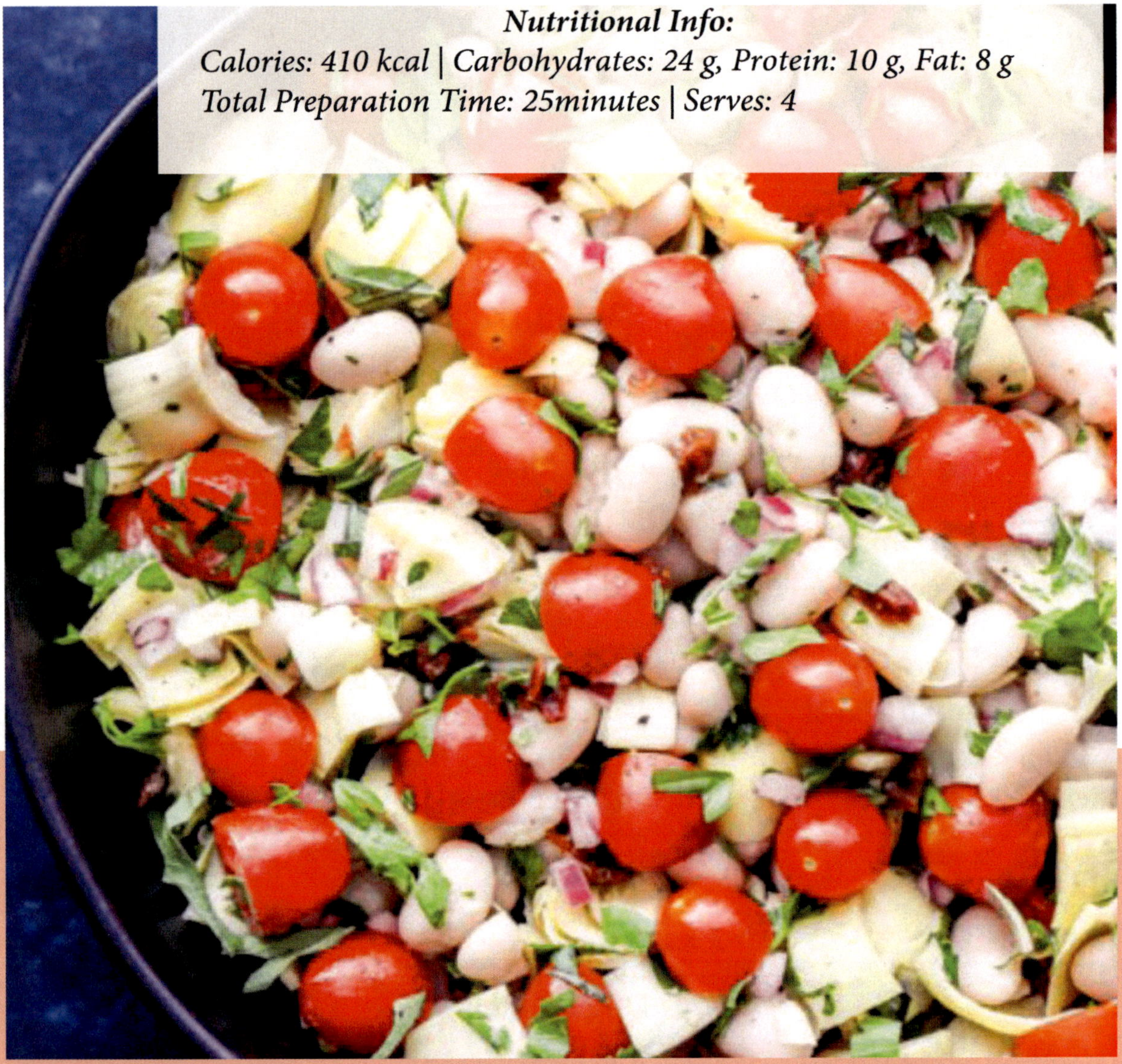

# *INGREDIENTS*

- *3 garlic cloves, minced*
- *Pinch of freshly ground black pepper*
- *2 jars of organic white beans in water without salt, drained*
- *6 medium tomatoes, chopped*
- *4 fresh artichokes*
- *1 leek, chopped*
- *1 tsp. of sea salt, to taste*
- *2 tsp. of extra virgin olive oil*
- *2 tsp. of freshly squeezed lemon juice*

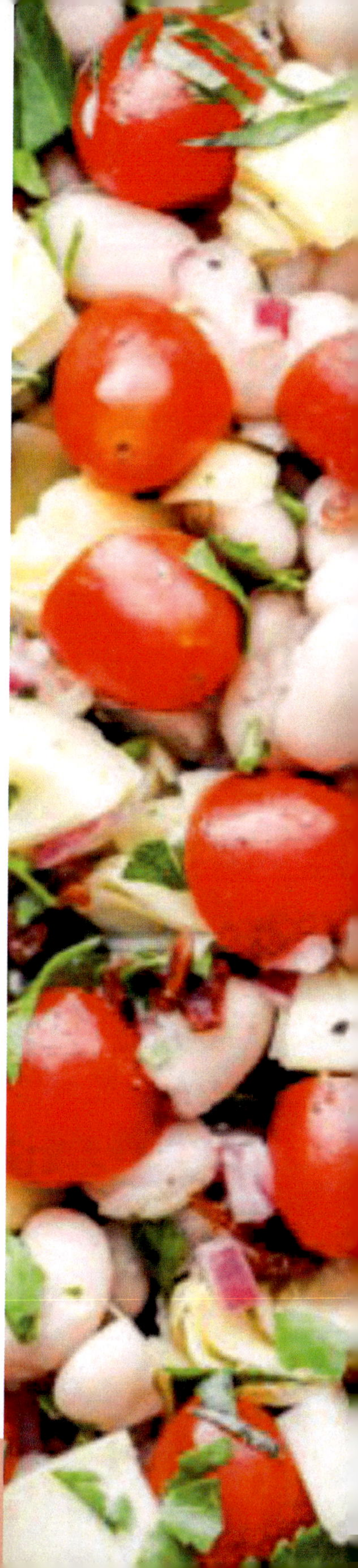

# *DIRECTIONS*

1. Rinse the artichokes under cold water.
2. Cut 1 inch off the top of the artichoke and trim the stem.
3. Remove the petals and squeeze the lemon juice on them.
4. Cut in half, lengthwise, and then in quarters.
5. Add the oil to the pan and place it over medium heat.
6. Add the garlic and stir fry for 60 seconds, until golden.
7. Then, add the artichoke quarters, a pinch of salt, chopped leek, and sauté for a few minutes.
8. Then, add the tomatoes, salt, and drained white beans.
9. Cover with the lid and cook for 18-20 minutes over medium heat, stirring occasionally.
10. Remove from the heat.
11. Serve and enjoy!

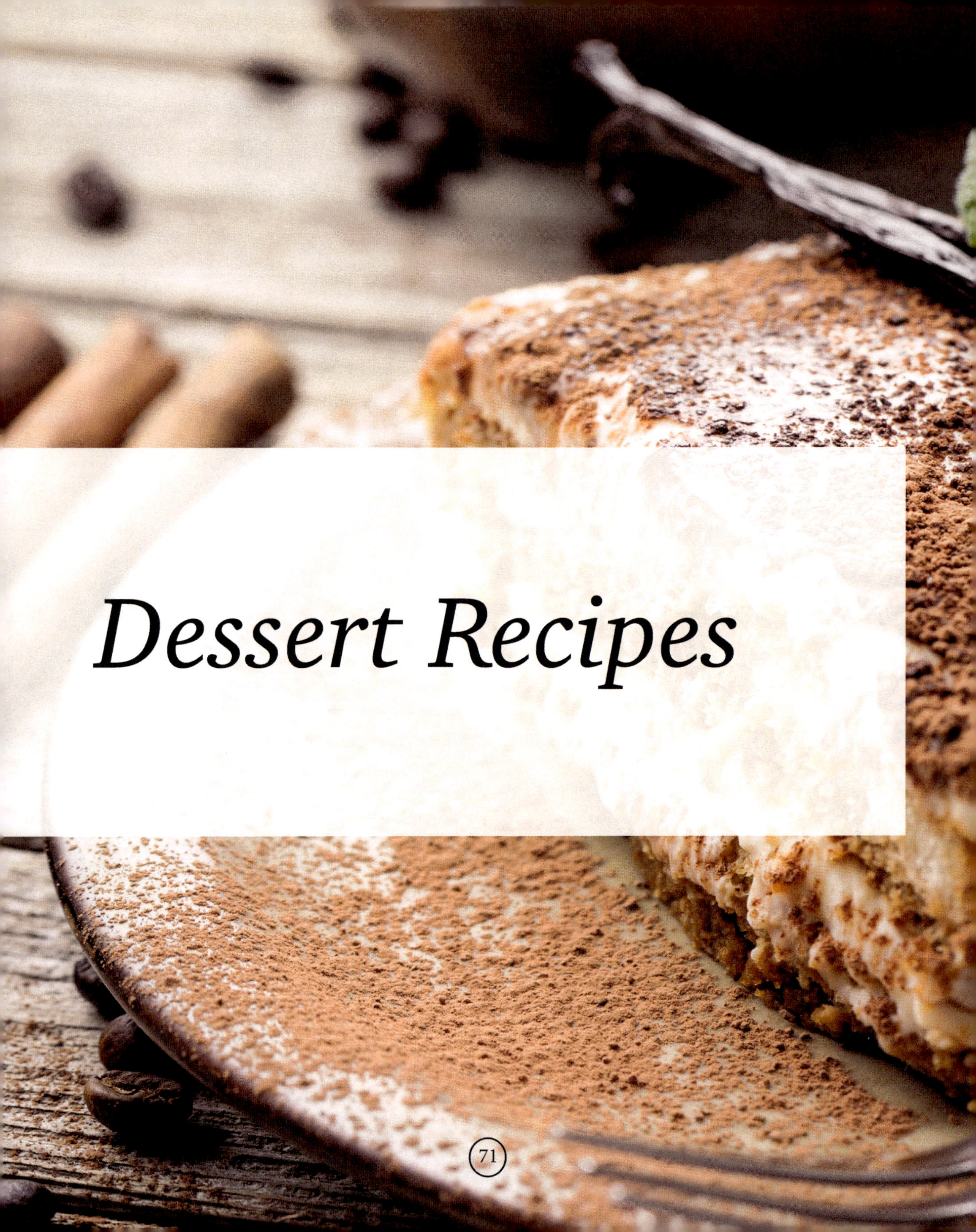

# Dessert Recipes

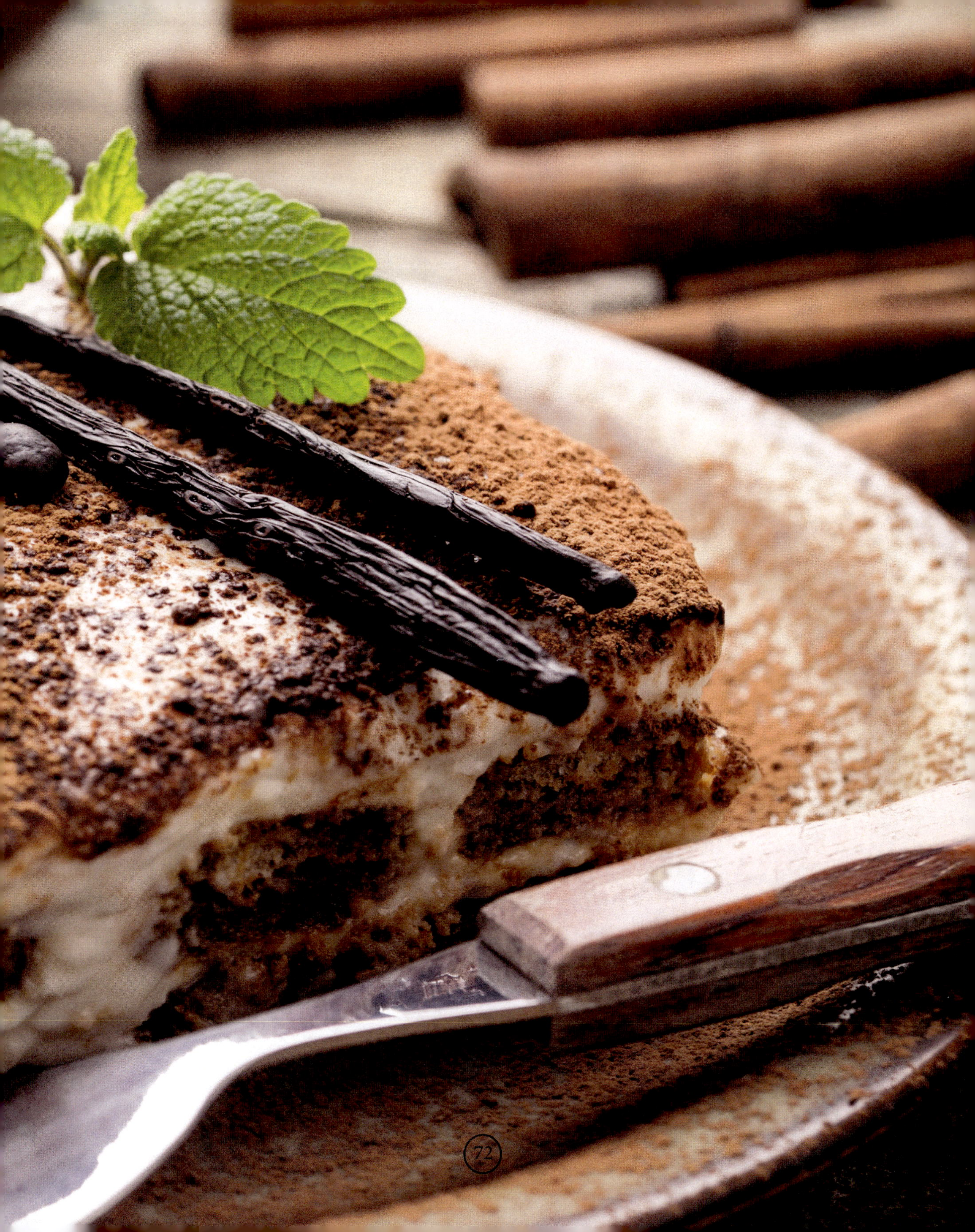

# *Strawberry-Melon Summer Salad*

LOVE'S HOLISTIC NUTRITION

***Nutritional Info:***

*Calories: 100 kcal | Carbohydrates: 3.3 g | Protein: 22.7 g | Fat: 0.4 g*

*Total Preparation Time: 10 minutes | Serves: 1*

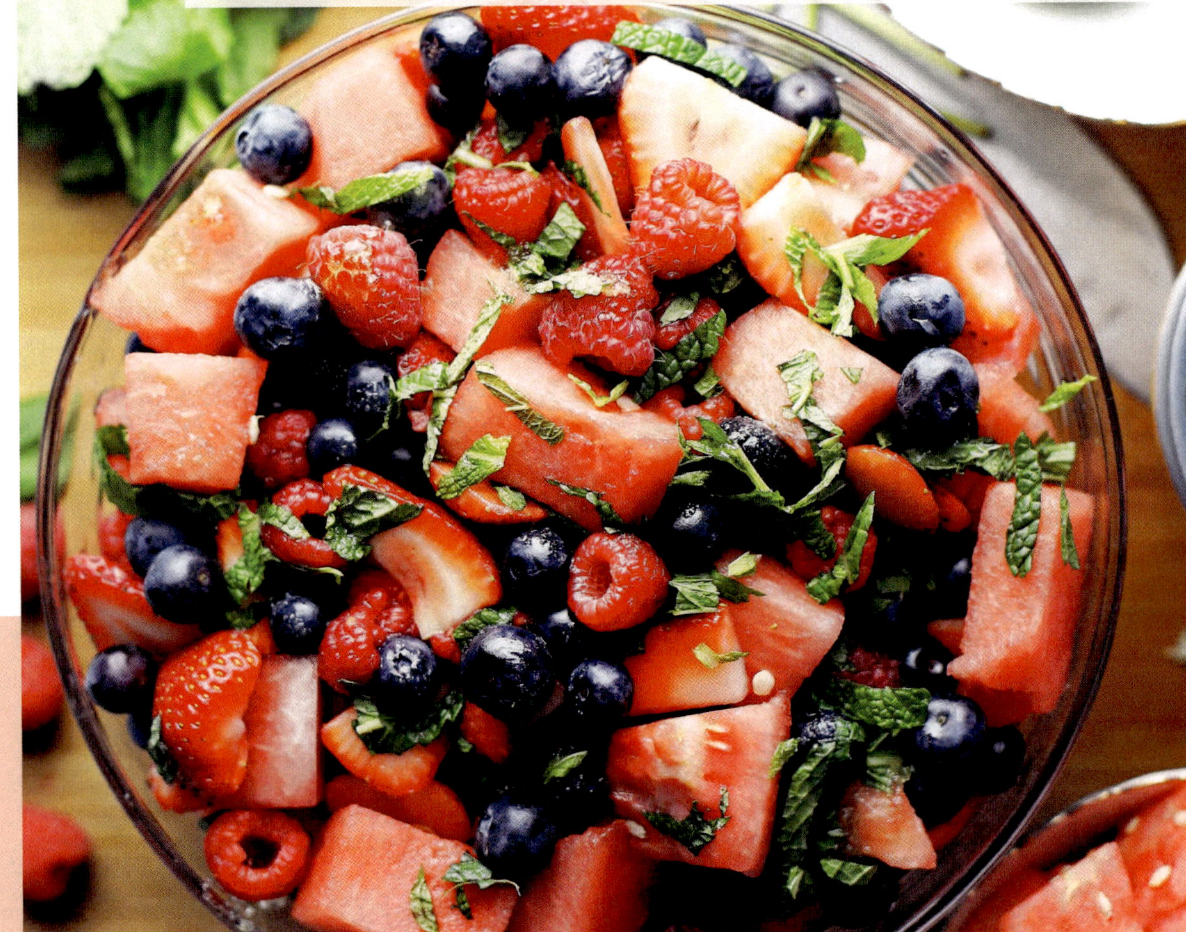

# INGREDIENTS

- *2 cups of fresh strawberries, halved*
- *3 tsp. of honey*
- *2 cups of watermelon*
- *2 cups of cantaloupe*
- *1 tsp. of fresh lemon juice*
- *1 cup of fresh lemon yogurt*

# DIRECTIONS

1. Mix the honey, lemon yogurt, and lemon juice in a salad bowl, until smooth.
2. Gently fold in the watermelon, cantaloupe, and strawberries.
3. Toss the fruit to coat.
4. Serve and enjoy!

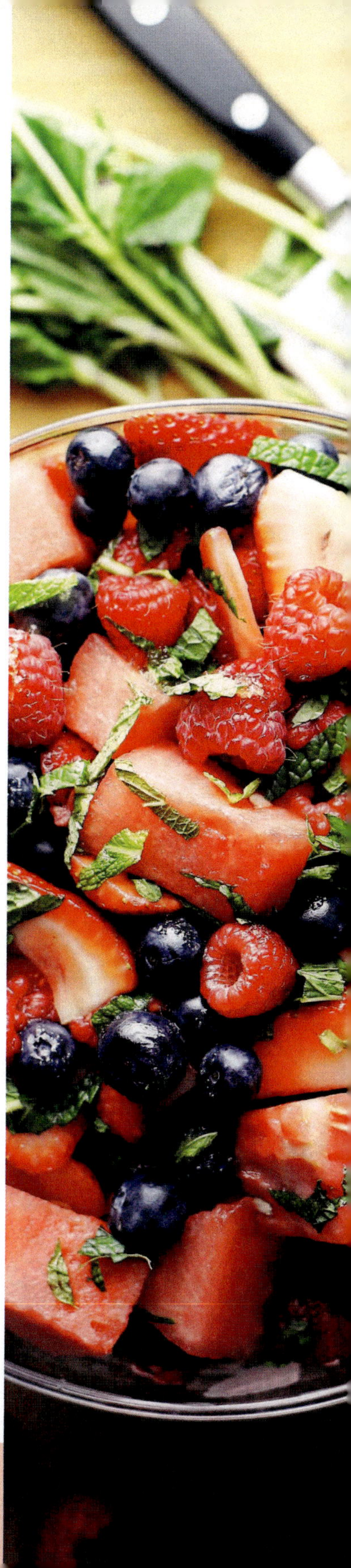

# Honey Lime Fruit Salad

**Nutritional Info:**
*Calories: 115 kcal | Carbohydrates: 22.3 g | Protein: 2.4 g | Fat: 3.3 g*
*Total Preparation Time: 20 minutes | Serves: 8*

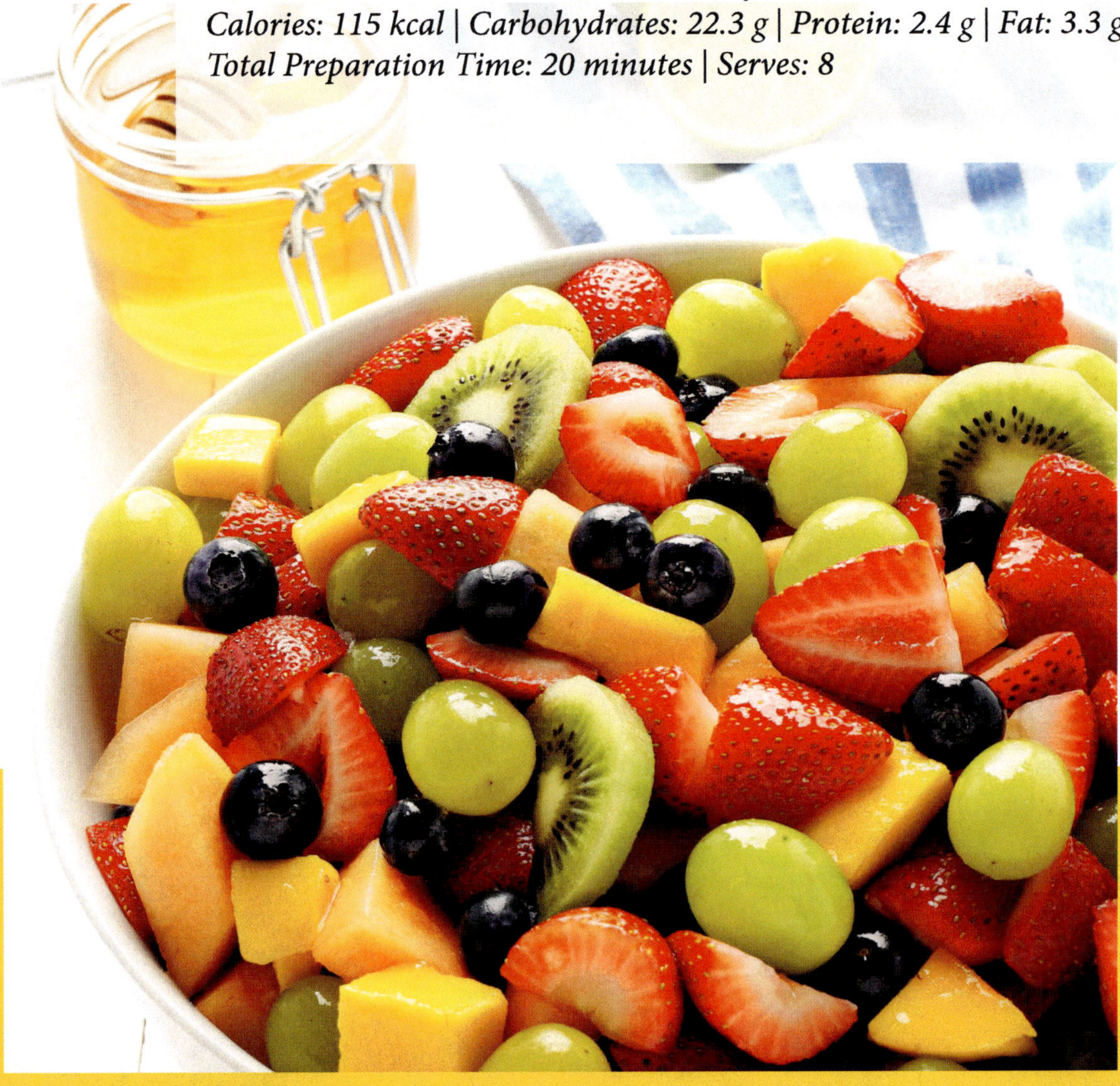

# INGREDIENTS

- *½ lb. of fresh blueberries*
- *2 tbsp. of honey*
- *1 fresh lime (for juice)*
- *⅓ cup of pine nuts*
- *2 large bananas, sliced*
- *16 oz. of fresh strawberries, sliced*

# DIRECTIONS

1. Place the bananas slices, strawberries slices, and fresh blueberries in the ceramic bowl.
2. Drizzle 2 tbsp. honey and the lime juice over the fruit.
3. Mix well to combine.
4. Sprinkle the pine nuts on top to garnish.
5. Serve and enjoy!

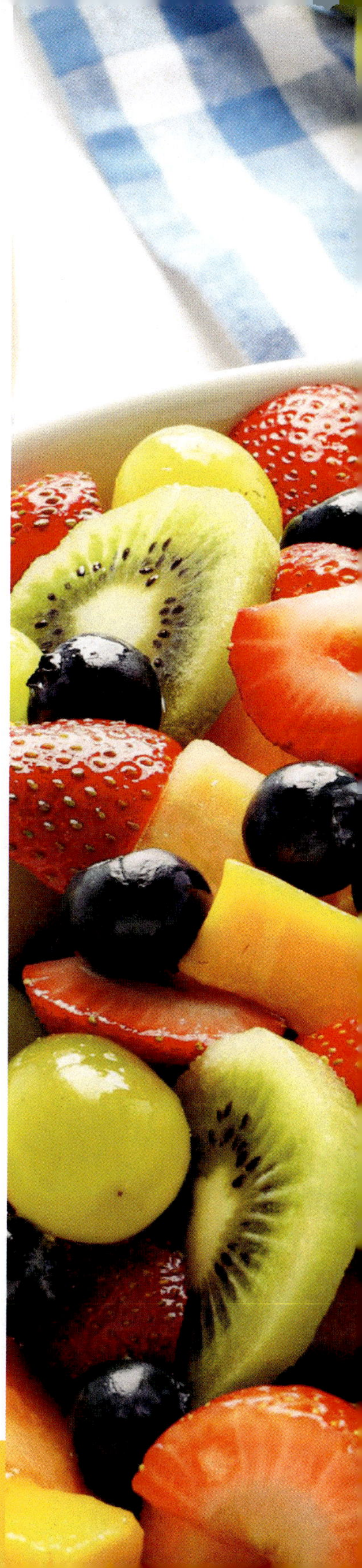

# *Tropical Island Fruit Salad*

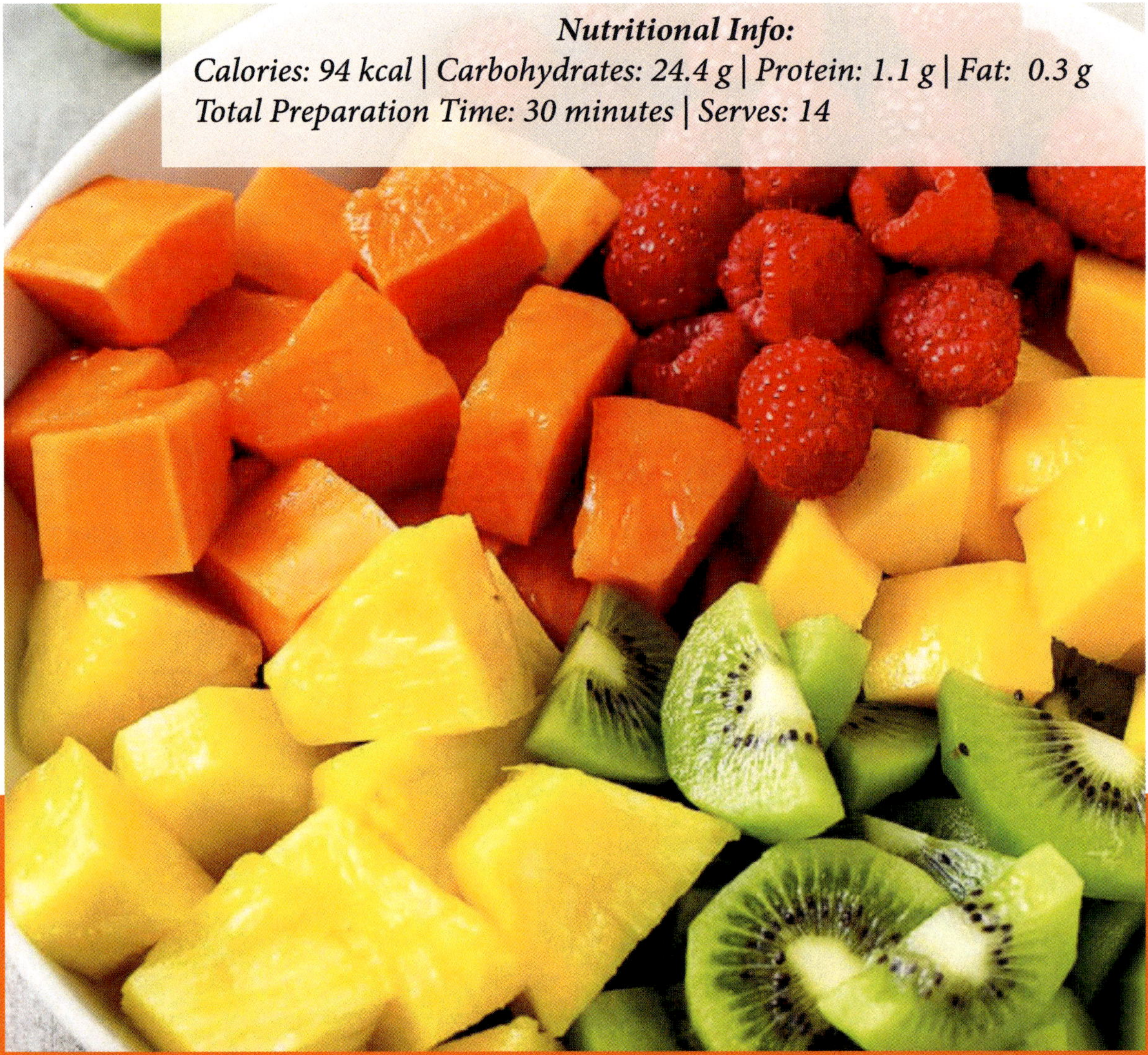

***Nutritional Info:***

*Calories: 94 kcal | Carbohydrates: 24.4 g | Protein: 1.1 g | Fat: 0.3 g*

*Total Preparation Time: 30 minutes | Serves: 14*

# *INGREDIENTS*

- *2 medium-sized mangos- peeled, pitted, and cubed*
- *3 medium-sized bananas, sliced*
- *1 small pineapple, peeled and cubed*
- *2 medium-sized papaya- halved lengthwise, seeded, peeled, and cubed*

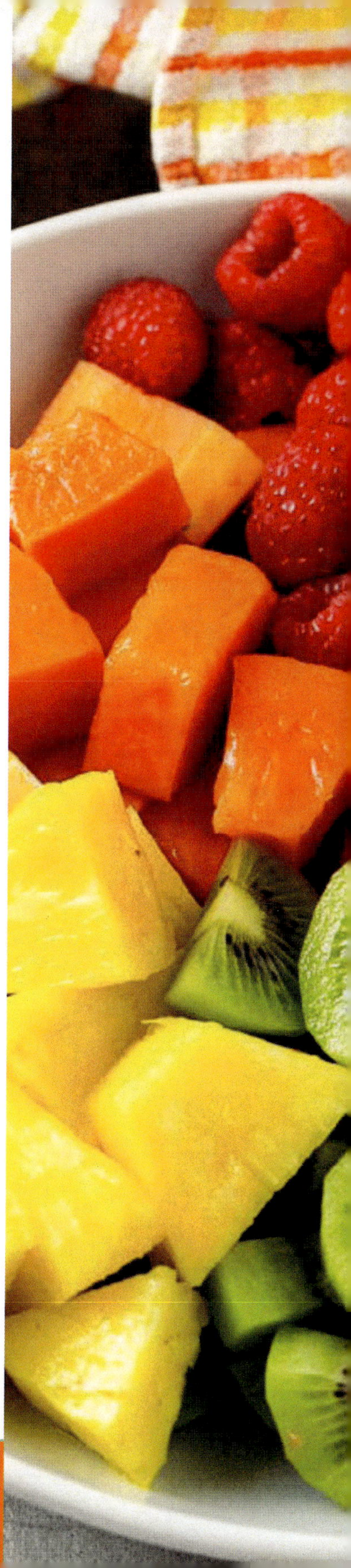

# *DIRECTIONS*

1. In a large ceramic bowl, and add all of the ingredients to the bowl.
2. Toss them well until combined.
3. Transfer the salad onto serving plates.
4. Serve and enjoy!

# Fruit Cocktail

**Nutritional Info:**

*Calories: 209 kcal | Carbohydrates: 38.3 g | Protein: 1.5 g | Fat: 0.6 g*
*Total Preparation Time: 22 minutes | Serves: 4*

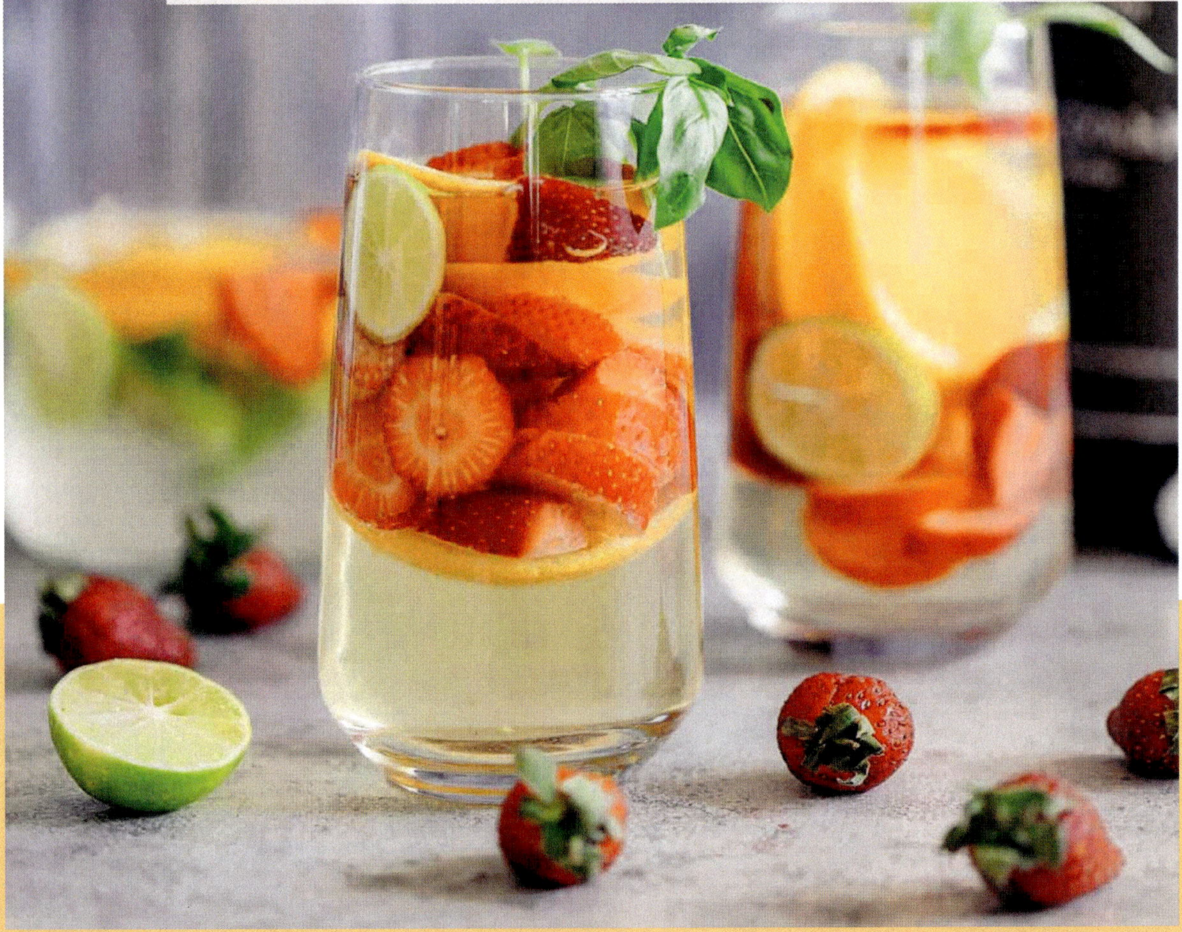

# *INGREDIENTS*

- *⅓ cup of white sugar*
- *1 pint of fresh strawberries, hulled and halved*
- *1 tbsp. of fresh mint, chopped*
- *½ cup of cantaloupes, bite-sized and cubed*
- *1 cup of seedless green grapes, halved*
- *1 ¼ cups white grape juice*

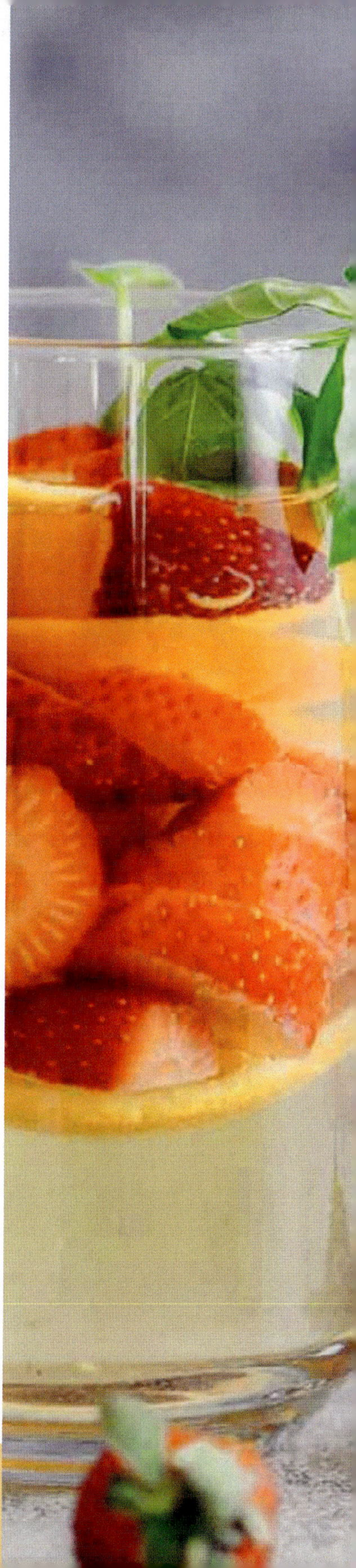

# *DIRECTIONS*

1. Place the saucepan over medium heat.
2. Combine the white grape juice and sugar.
3. Bring to a boil and stir until the sugar dissolves.
4. Turn off the burner and add the mint.
5. Set aside.
6. In a large bowl, combine the cantaloupe, grapes, and strawberries.
7. Pour the white grape juice mixture over the fruit.
8. Toss the fruit in the white grape mixture until well-coated.
9. Cover and refrigerate for up to 8 hours.
10. Serve and enjoy!

# *Fruit Salad for Easter Sunday*

LOVE'S HOLISTIC NUTRITION

***Nutritional Info:***

*Calories: 146 kcal | Carbohydrates: 34 g | Protein: 4.1 g | Fat: 0.5 g*

*Total Preparation Time: 20 minutes | Serves: 8*

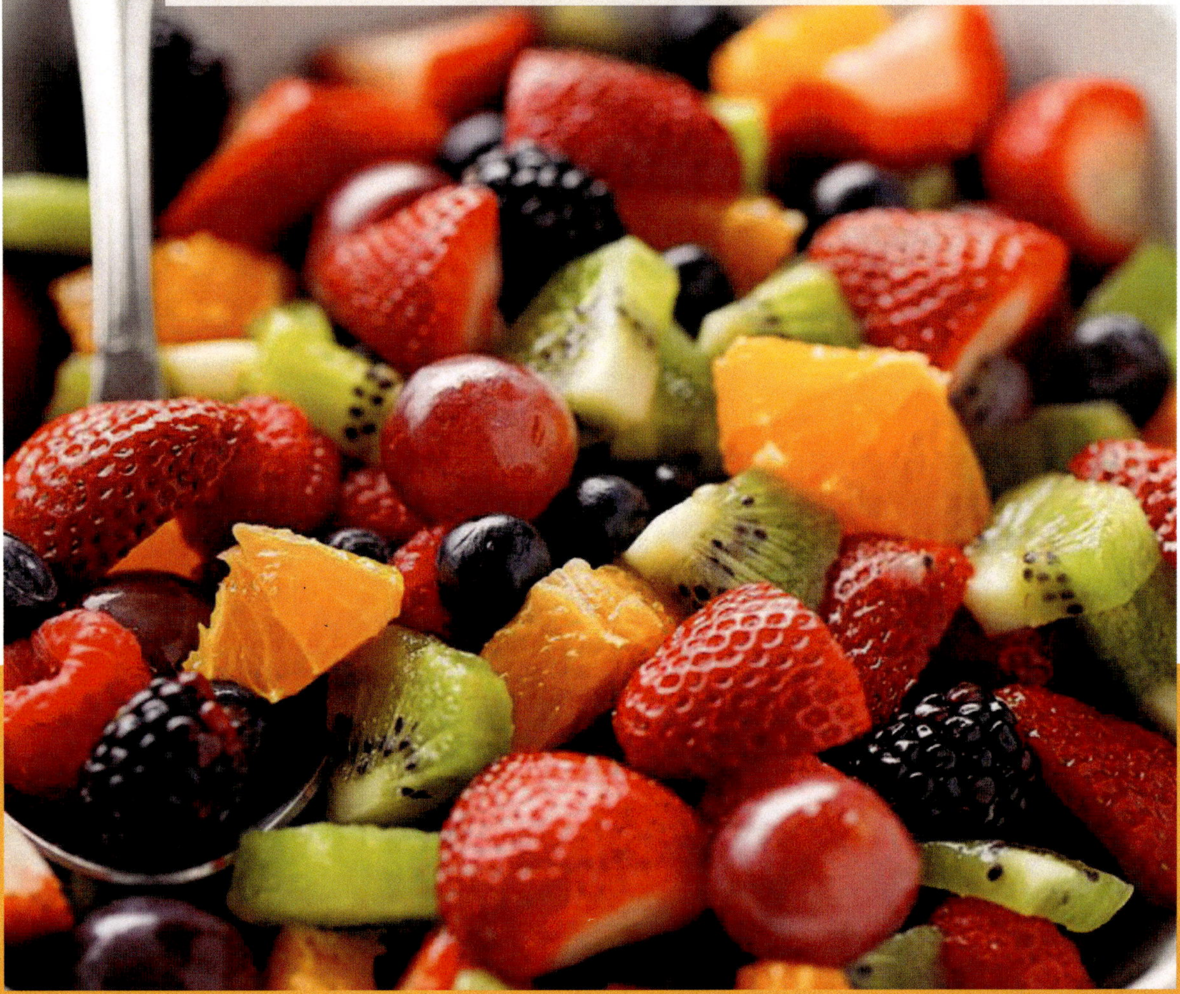

# *INGREDIENTS*

- *1 medium apple, cored and chopped*
- *15 oz. of pineapple chunks*
- *1 cup of red grapes*
- *2 cups of lemon yogurt, fresh*
- *2 kiwi fruit, peeled and diced*
- *1 Granny Smith apple, chopped*
- *1 cup of fresh blueberries*

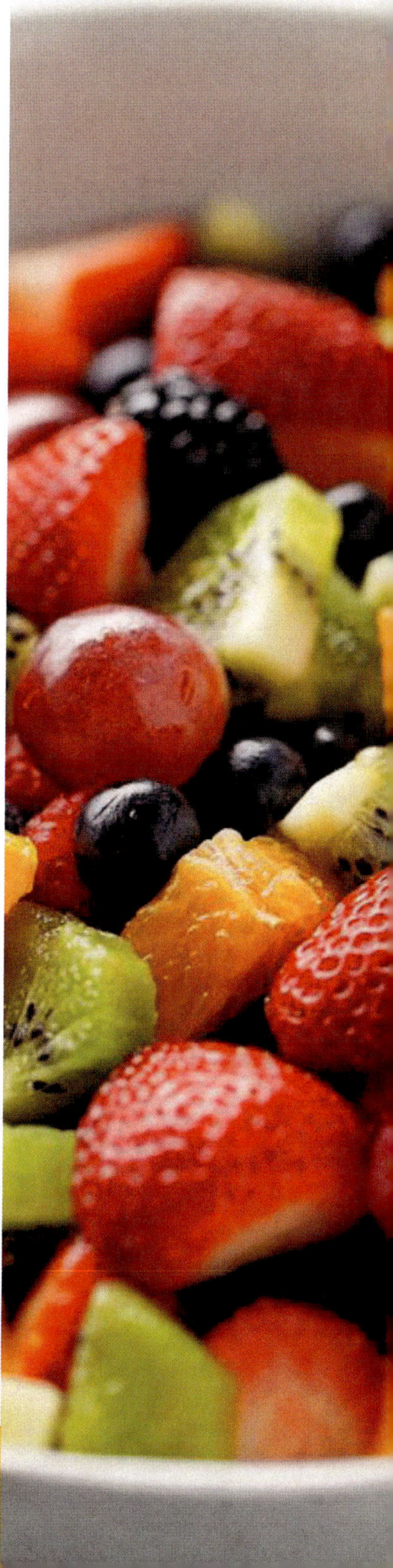

# *DIRECTIONS*

1. Mix the strawberries, blueberries, apples, kiwi fruit, pineapple chunks, red grapes, and lemon yogurt together in a bowl.
2. Serve and enjoy!

# *Lime Basil Pie*

***Nutritional Info:***
*Calories: 215 kcal | Carbohydrates: 18.2 g | Protein: 4.7 g | Fat: 10.4 g*
*Total Preparation Time: 30 minutes | Serves: 8*

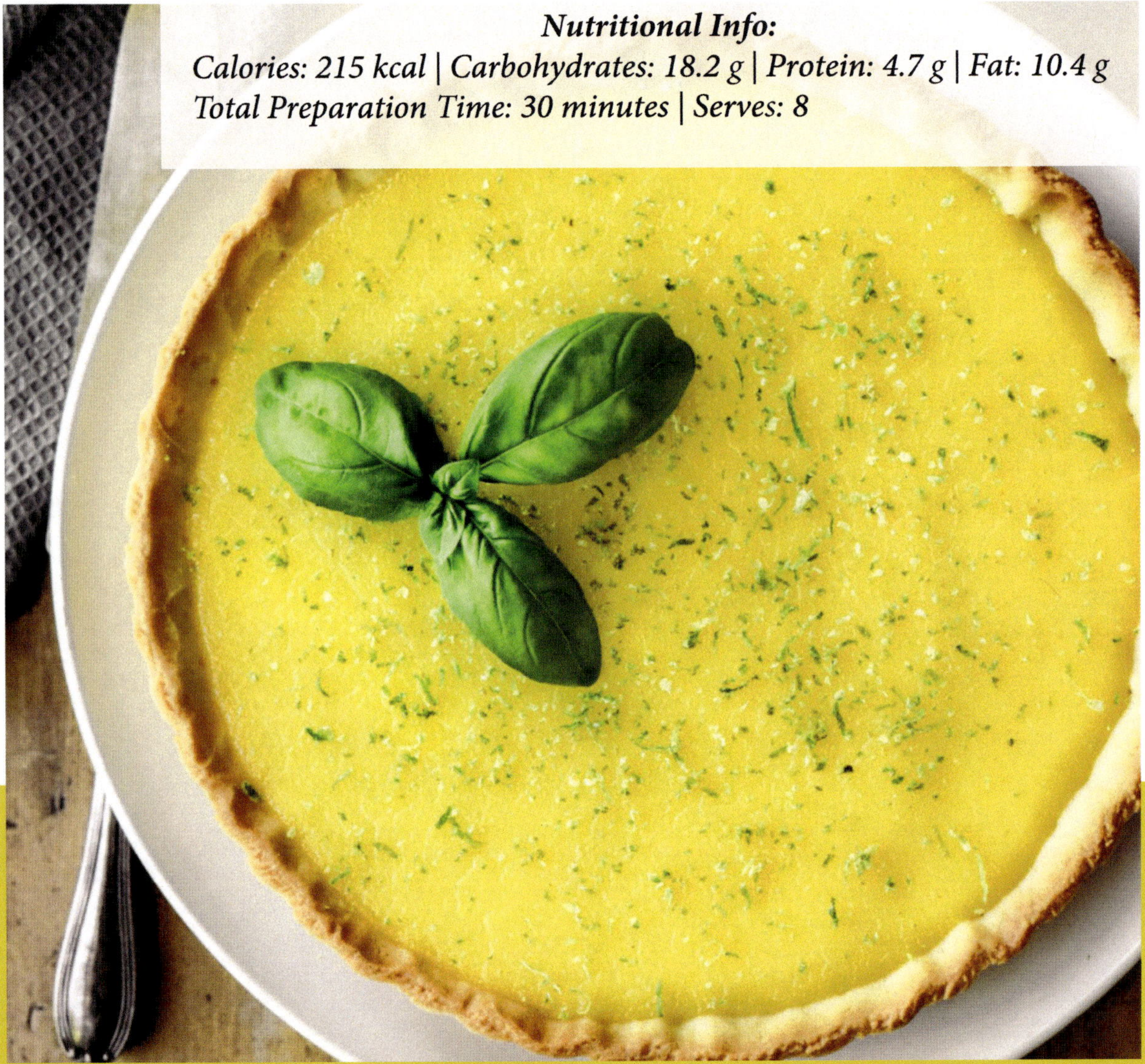

# *INGREDIENTS*

- *8 oz. of reduced-fat cream cheese*
- *14 oz. of fat-free sweetened condensed milk*
- *Sweetened whipped cream, optional*
- *1 tbsp. of grated lime zest*
- *¼ cup of fresh basil, chopped*
- *1 reduced-fat graham cracker crust (9 in.)*
- *2 large egg yolks*
- *½ cup lime juice, fresh*

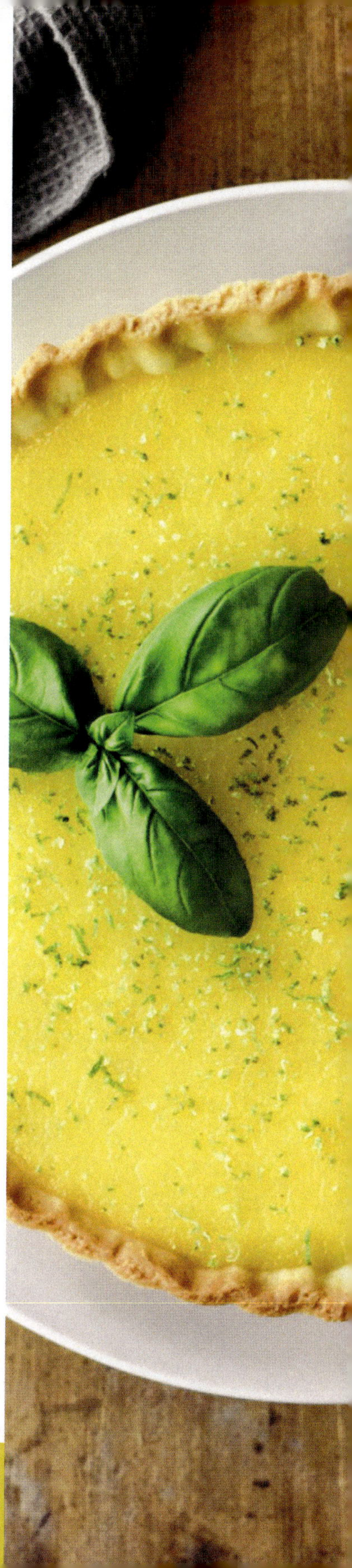

# *DIRECTIONS*

1. Preheat the oven to 325°F.
2. In a large mixing basin, beat the cream cheese until smooth; add the milk, gradually.
3. Beat in the lime zest, lime juice, and egg yolks, just until combined.
4. Combine with the basil.
5. Pour into the prepared crust.
6. Bake for 17 minutes until the middle is completely set.
7. Allow 1 hour to cool on a wire rack.
8. Refrigerate for 2 hours (at least) before serving.
9. Garnish with whipped cream, if preferred.
10. Serve and enjoy!

# *Bacon Chocolate Chip Cheesecake Blondies*

***Nutritional Info:***

*Calories: 145 kcal | Carbohydrates: 14.1 g | Protein: 2.5 g | Fat: 21.2 g*
*Total Preparation Time: 1 hr, 15 minutes | Serves: 16*

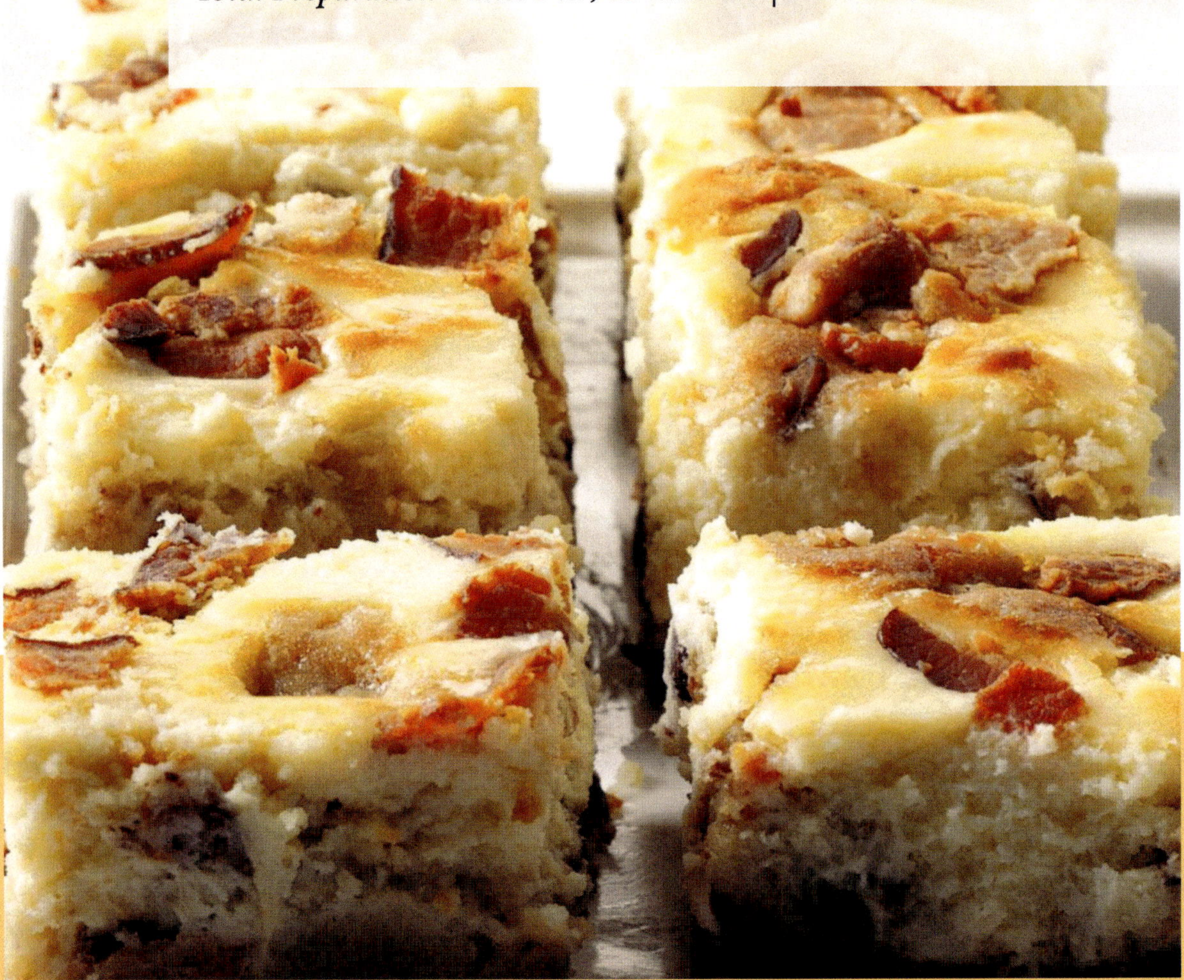

# *INGREDIENTS*

- *1 cup of butter, softened*
- *¾ cup of white sugar*
- *¾ cup of brown sugar*
- *2 large eggs*
- *2¼ cups of all-purpose flour*
- *1 tsp. of salt*
- *¾ cup of milk*
- *1 tsp. of baking soda*
- *2 cups of semisweet chocolate chips*
- *8 oz. of cream cheese, softened*
- *1 cup of sugar*
- *2 tsp. of vanilla extract*
- *8 bacon strips, cooked and crumbled*
- *1 tsp. of vanilla extract*

# *DIRECTIONS*

1. Preheat the oven to 375°F.
2. Wrap the foil around a 9-inch square baking pan, allowing the ends to extend up the edges.
3. Grease the foil.
4. Set aside 1/4 of the bacon crumbles for the topping.
5. Place the cream, butter, and sugars in a large ceramic bowl and mix until light and creamy; incorporate the eggs and vanilla extract.
6. In a separate basin, whisk together the flour, salt, and baking soda
7. Gradually incorporate flour mixture into a creamed mixture.
8. Combine the chocolate chips and bacon in a separate bowl.
9. Expand half of the dough into the base of the ready pan.
10. To make the cheesecake layer, whisk the cream cheese and sugar until smooth in a large mixing basin.
11. Combine the eggs, milk, and vanilla extract in a mixing bowl; beat on a moderate speed, until combined.
12. Pour over the dough in prepared pan;space the remaining dough over the cheesecake layer with rounded tablespoons.
13. Bake for 41-44 minutes, or until golden brown.
14. Allow cooling in the pan on a wire rack. Refrigerate for four hours (at least) before cutting.
15. Garnish with the remaining bacon crumbles.
16. Divide into bars and remove from the pan using foil tongs
17. Serve and enjoy!

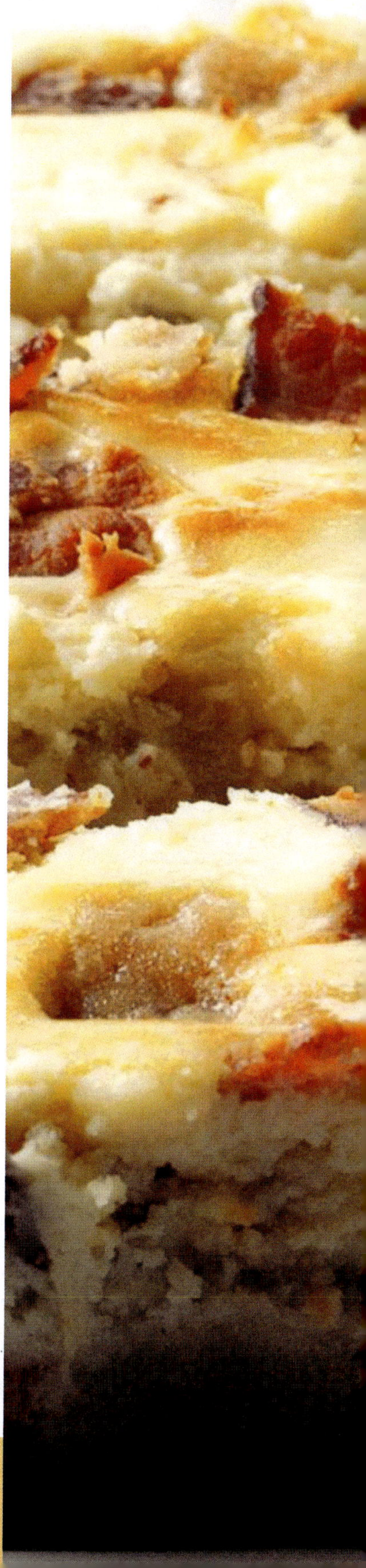

# *Red Curry Pandan Ice Cream*

LOVE'S HOLISTIC NUTRITION

**Nutritional Info:**

*Calories: 236 kcal | Carbohydrates: 15.9 g | Protein: 5.1 g | Fat: 19.4 g*
*Total Preparation Time: 50 minutes | Serves: 1*

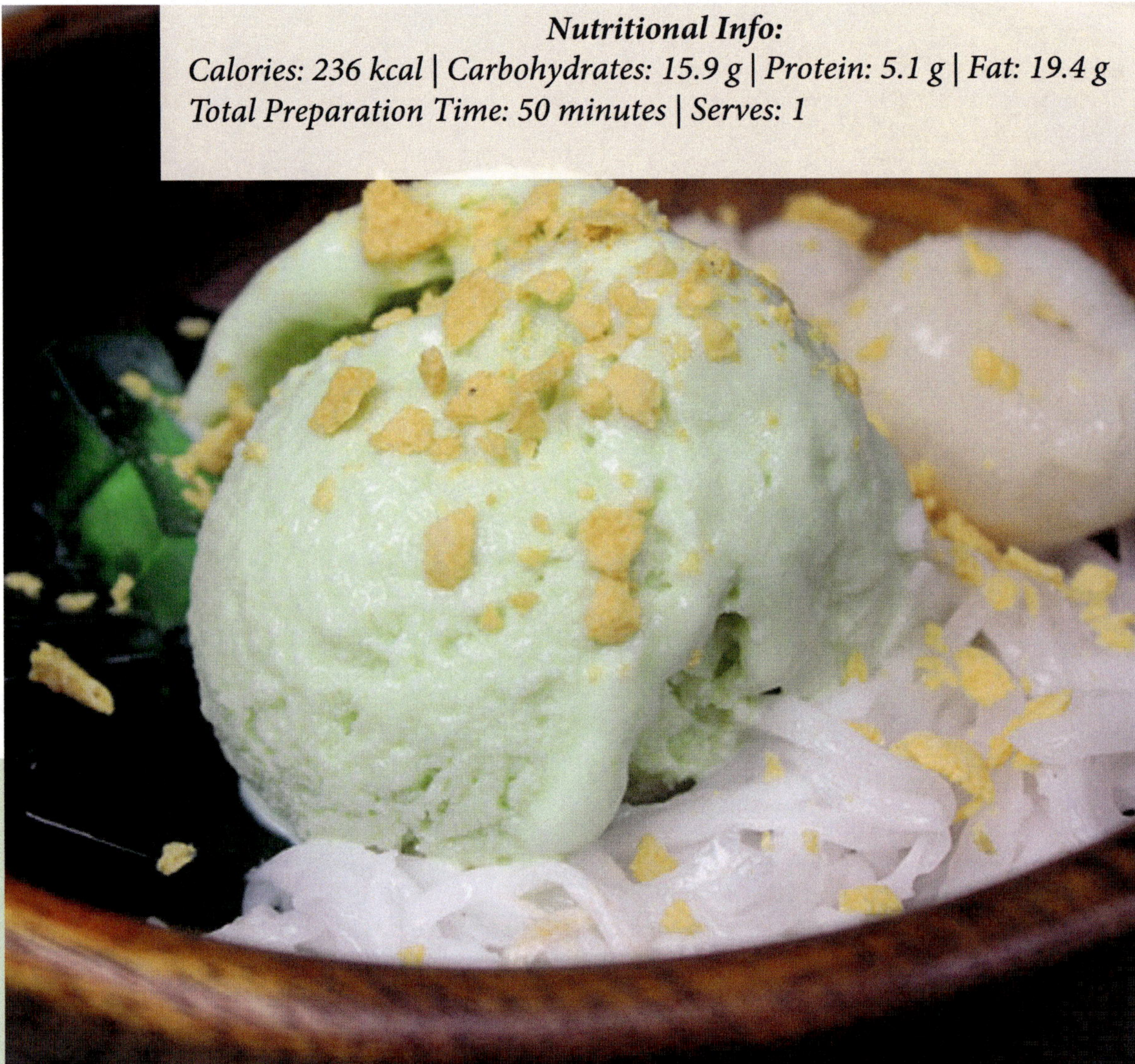

# *INGREDIENTS*

- *3 pandan leaves*
- *15 oz. of cream of coconut*
- *½ cups of heavy whipping cream*
- *1 drop of food color, green*
- *½ tsp. of red curry powder*
- *1 cup of fresh whole milk*

# *DIRECTIONS*

1. Combine the milk, pandan, and curry powder in a small saucepan.
2. Increase the heat until it boils.
3. Take the pan off of the heat.
4. Cover and steep for 30 minutes.
5. The panDan should be removed and discarded.
6. Combine the coconut cream, whipped cream, food coloring (if desired), and milk mixture in a blender.
7. Cover and pulse until completely smooth.
8. Fill the ice cream freezer cylinder 2/3 of the way.
9. Freeze, as directed.
10. Shift the ice cream to the freezer container and freeze for an additional 2-4 hours.
11. Serve and enjoy!

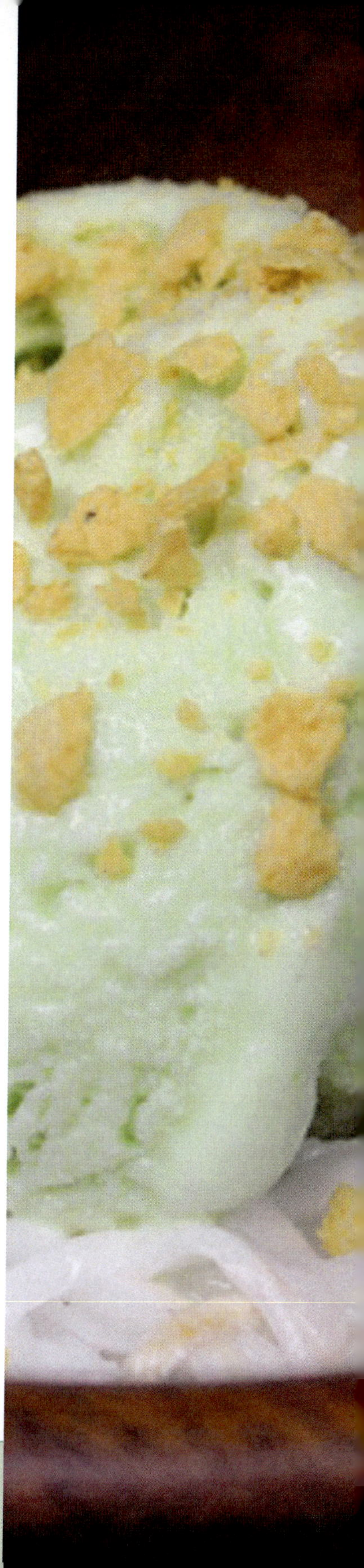

# *Salted Caramel & Dark Chocolate Figs*

***Nutritional Info:***

*Calories: 232 kcal | Carbohydrates: 13.1 g | Protein: 4.2 g | Fat: 15.9 g*

*Total Preparation Time: 30 minutes | Serves: 1*

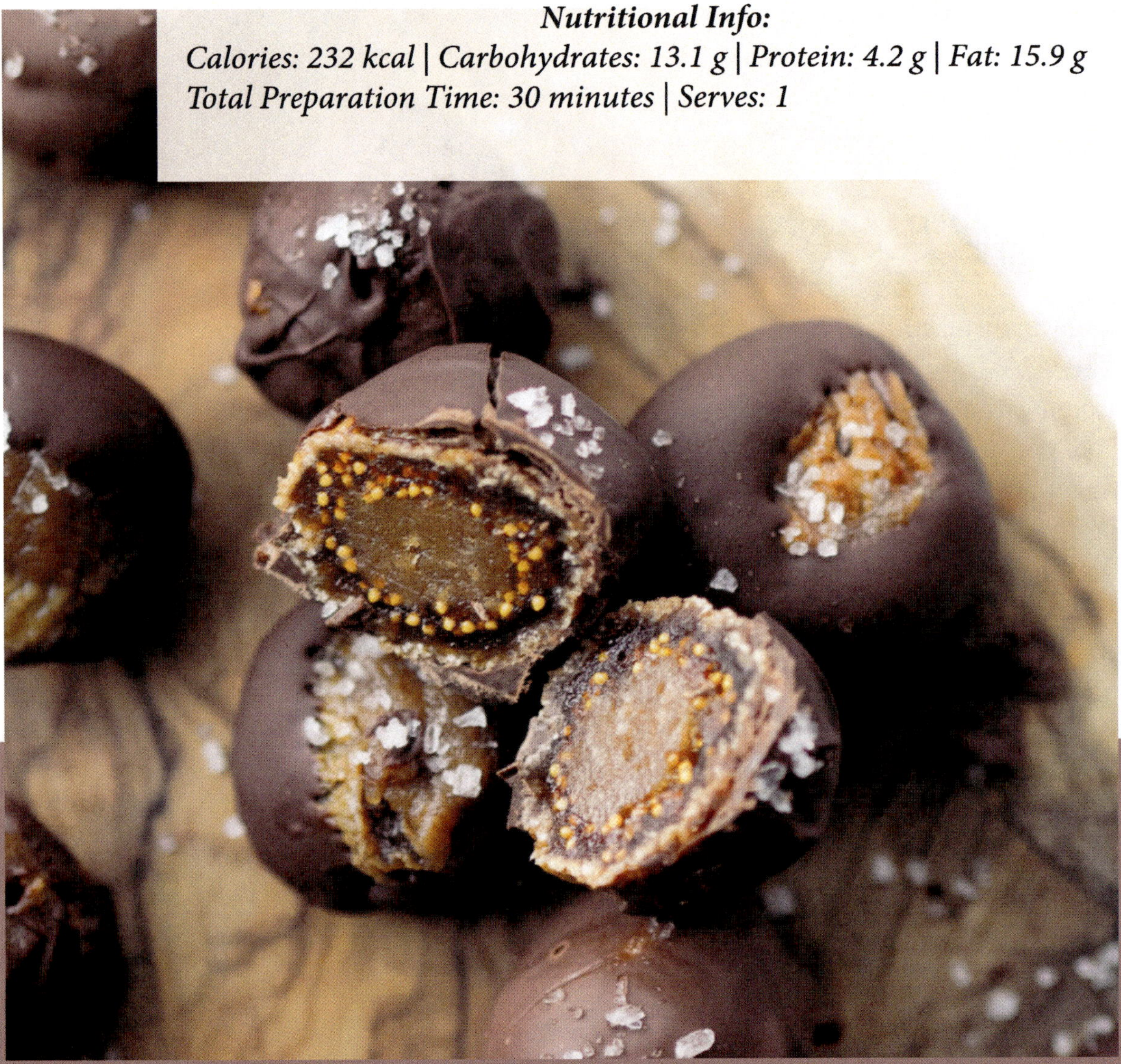

# INGREDIENTS

- *4 oz. of fresh goat cheese*
- *1 tsp. of honey*
- *11 oz. of Kraft caramel bits*
- *2 tbsp. of water*
- *⅓ cup cup of almonds, chopped*
- *Coarse sea salt*
- *½ cups of dark chocolate chips, softened*
- *12 dried figs*
- *1 tsp. balsamic vinegar*
- *12 large toothpicks*

# DIRECTIONS

1. Assemble the baking sheet by lining it with waxed paper and greasing it; set aside. Each fig should be pricked with a toothpick.
2. Each fig should have a ½ inch cut on the side.
3. In a small ceramic bowl, combine the cheese, honey, and vinegar.
4. Transfer to a large resealable plastic bag; cut a small hole in one of the bag's corners.
5. Fill the figs halfway with the cheese mixture.
6. In a microwave, melt the caramels and water; whisk until smooth.
7. Each fig should be dipped into caramel and turned to coat.
8. Arrange the figs in prepared pan and set aside until set.
9. Place the almonds in a small shallow bowl.
10. Soak the base third of each fig into melted chocolate and set aside any excess.
11. Indulge in almonds and season with salt.
12. Reintroduce to the pan; set aside until set.
13. Serve and enjoy!

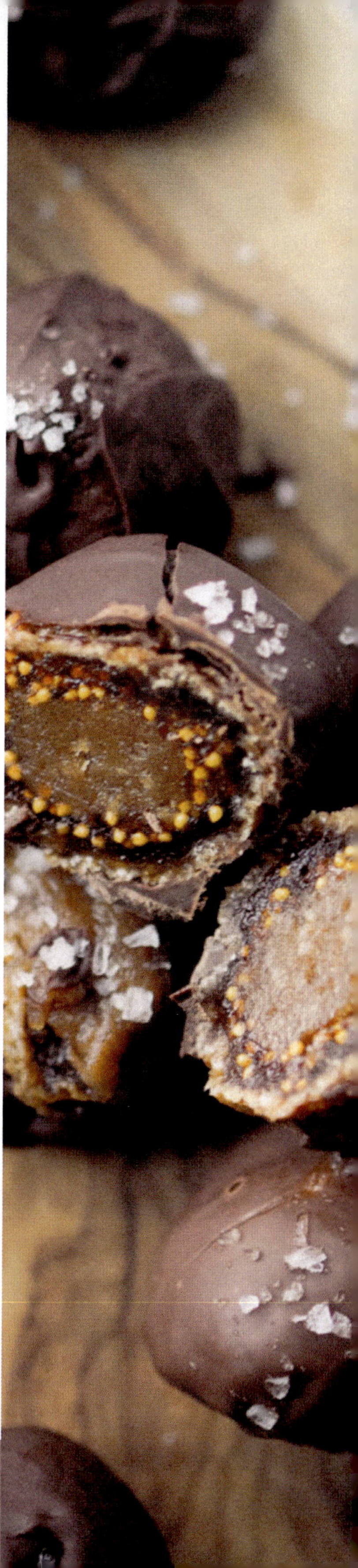

# *Olive Oil Cake*

LOVE'S HOLISTIC NUTRITION

***Nutritional Info:***

*Calories: 245 kcal | Carbohydrates: 13.1 g | Protein: 3.3g | Fat: 19.4 g*
*Total Preparation Time: 60 minutes | Serves: 16*

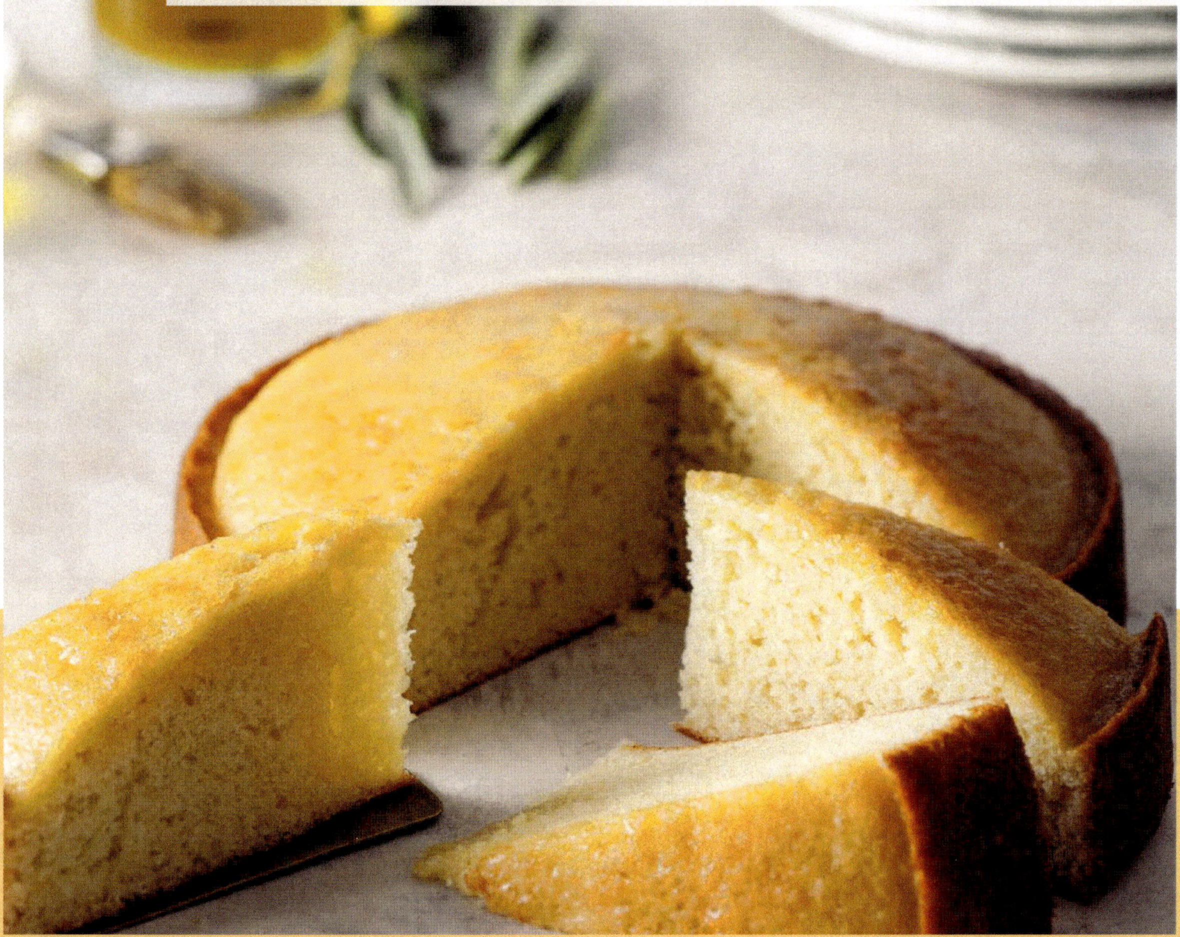

# *INGREDIENTS*

- *½ cups of sugar*
- *¾ cup of extra virgin olive oil*
- *1 tbsp. of grated orange zest*
- *¾ cups of all-purpose flour*
- *2 tsp. of baking powder*
- *½ tsp. of salt*
- *¾ cup of confectioners' sugar*
- *1/4 cup of orange juice*
- *Roasted almonds, chopped (optional)*
- *1 tsp. of vanilla extract*
- *3 large eggs*
- *½ cup of milk*
- *¾ cup of ground almonds*

# *DIRECTIONS*

1. Preheat the oven to 325°F.
2. Coat the 10-inch fluted pan with cooking spray and flour.
3. In a large ceramic bowl, beat the eggs for 3 minutes on high speed, adding the sugar gradually.
4. Beat until thick and lemon-colored.
5. Beat in the oil, slowly.
6. Combine the ground almonds, milk, orange zest, and vanilla extract in a mixing bowl.
7. In the other bowl, beat the flour with baking powder and salt.
8. Incorporate the flour mixture into the egg mixture.
9. Spread the batter evenly in the prepared pan.
10. Bake for 46-49 minutes, or until a toothpick inserted near the middle comes out clean.
11. Allow 15 minutes for cooling in the pan before transferring to a wire rack to cool entirely.
12. Whisk the sugar and orange juice in a small bowl until it reaches a dripping consistency for the icing.
13. Drizzle the glaze over the cake top.
    *Optional: Sprinkle with almonds, if desired.*
14. Serve and enjoy!

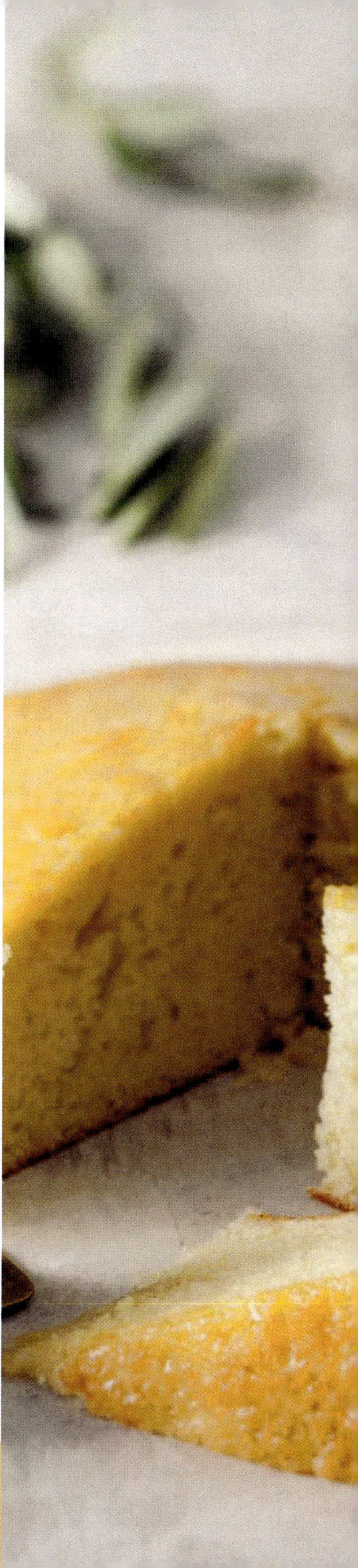

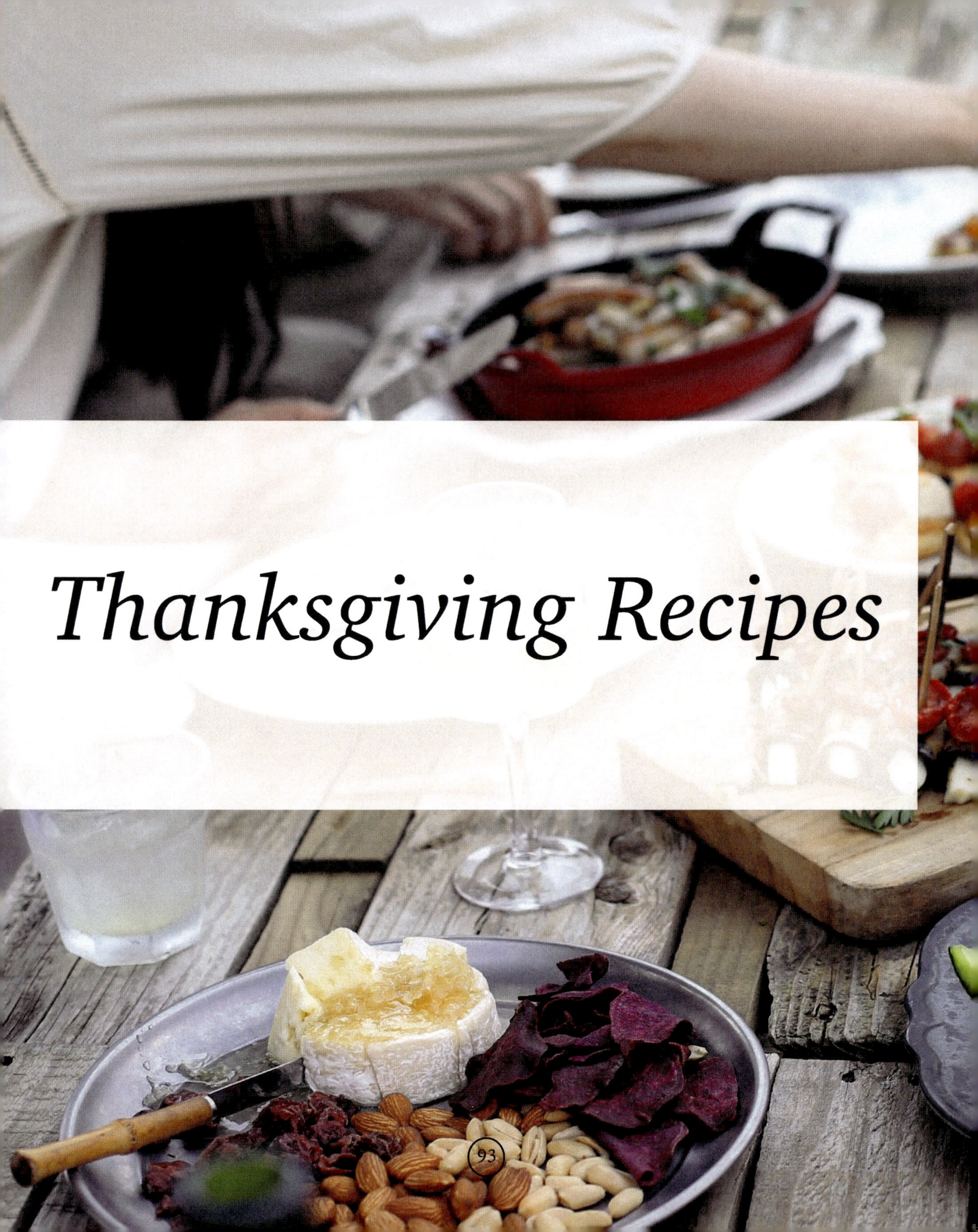

# Thanksgiving Recipes

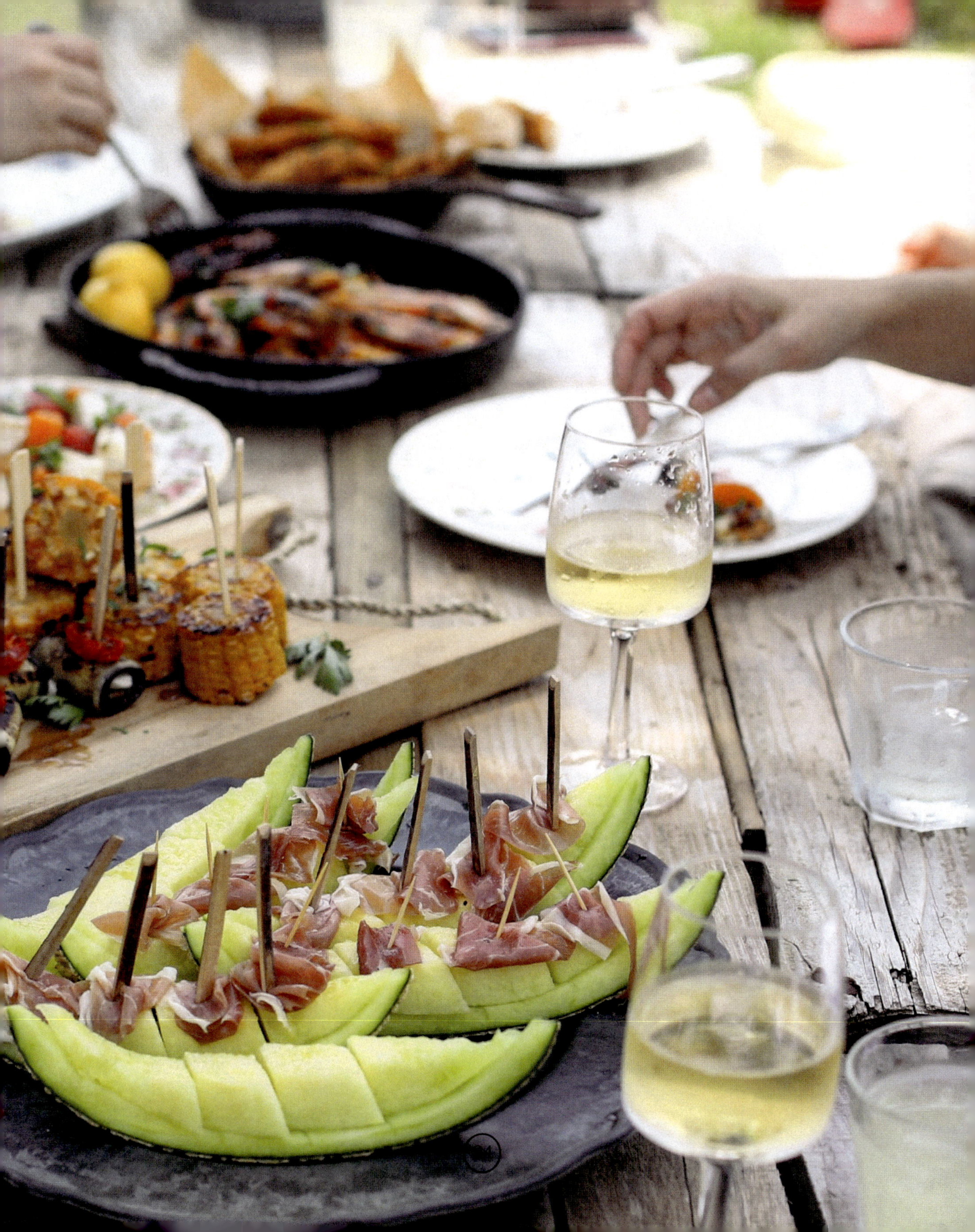

# *Perfect Roast Turkey*

***Nutritional Info:***

*Calories: 50 kcal | Carbohydrates: 1 g | Protein: 11 g | Fat: 9 g*
*Total Preparation Time: 3 hrs, 20 minutes | Serves: 8*

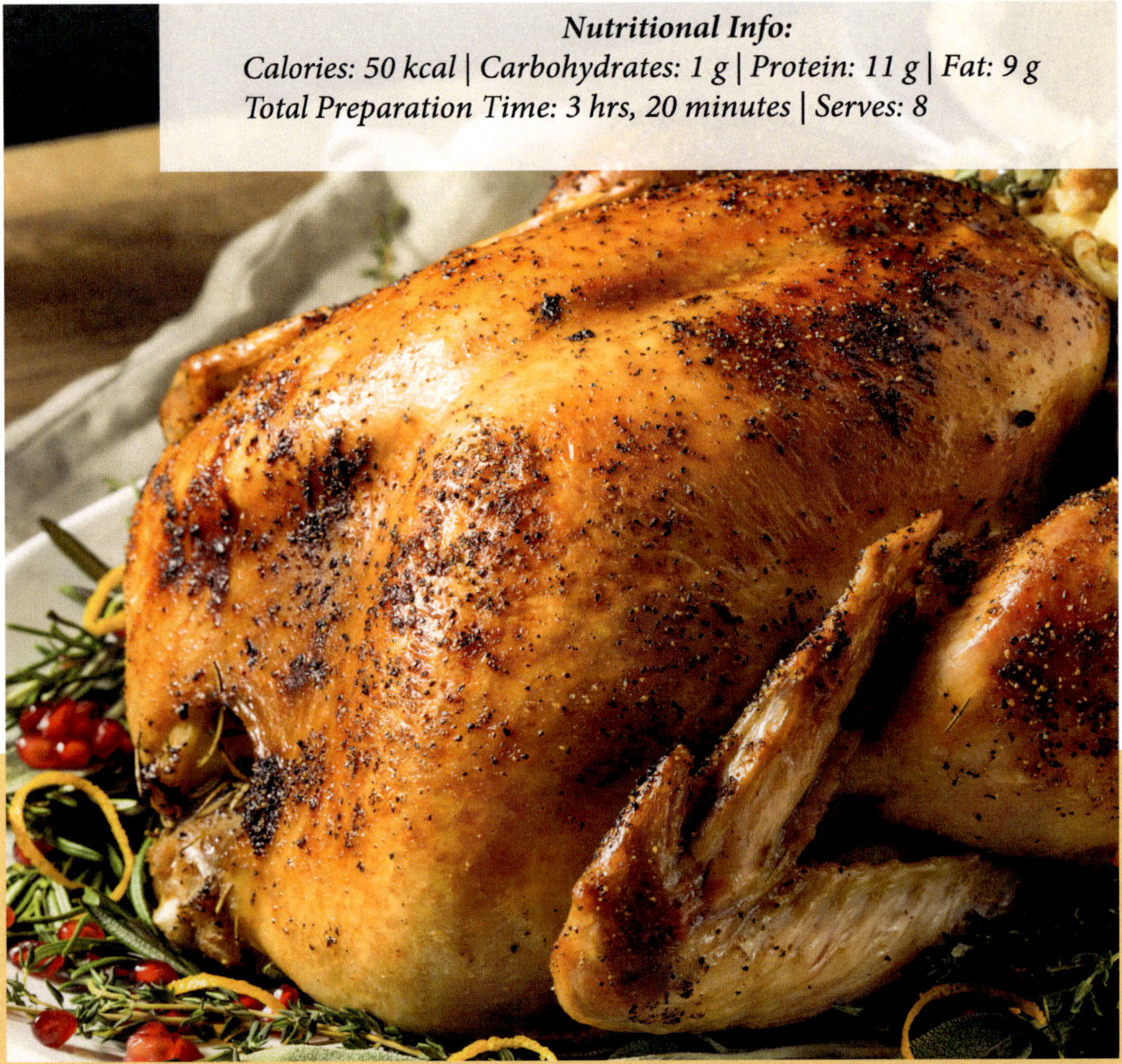

# INGREDIENTS

- *14 lb. unsalted butter*
- *1 fresh lemon, zested and juiced*
- *1 tsp. fresh thyme leaves, chopped*
- *1 fresh turkey (about 12 lb)*
- *2 small bunches of fresh thyme*
- *Kosher salt to taste*
- *1 red onion, chopped*
- *1 garlic clove, halved chopped*
- *1 whole lemon, halved*
- *Freshly ground black pepper*

# DIRECTIONS

1. Preheat the oven to 350°F.
2. In a small saucepan, melt the butter.
3. Add the lemon zest, thyme, and lemon juice to the butter mixture.
4. Place aside.
5. Remove the giblets from the turkey and thoroughly wash them inside and out.
6. Remove any excess fat and pinfeathers from the exterior and dry.
7. Place the turkey in a big roasting pan.
8. Season the inside of the turkey cavity well with salt and pepper.
9. Fill the cavity with a sprig of thyme, half lemon, quartered onion, and a clove of garlic.
10. Brush the butter mixture around the outside of the turkey and season with salt and pepper.
11. String the legs together and tuck the wing tips beneath the turkey's body.
12. Roast the turkey for approximately 2½ hours, or until the juices flow clear when the leg and thigh are separated.
13. Transfer the turkey to a chopping board.
14. Remove the aluminum foil and set aside for 20 minutes to rest.
15. Slice the turkey.
16. Serve and enjoy!

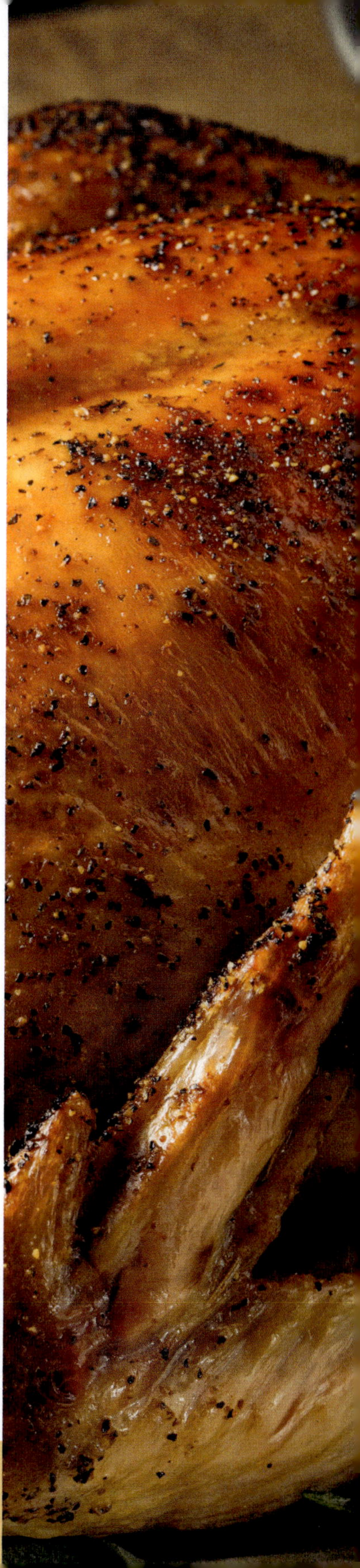

# Oven-Baked Chicken

Love's Holistic Nutrition

***Nutritional Info:***

*Calories: 780 kcal | Carbohydrates: 59 g | Protein: 63 g | Fat: 31 g*

*Total Preparation Time: 1 hr, 55 minutes | Serves: 4*

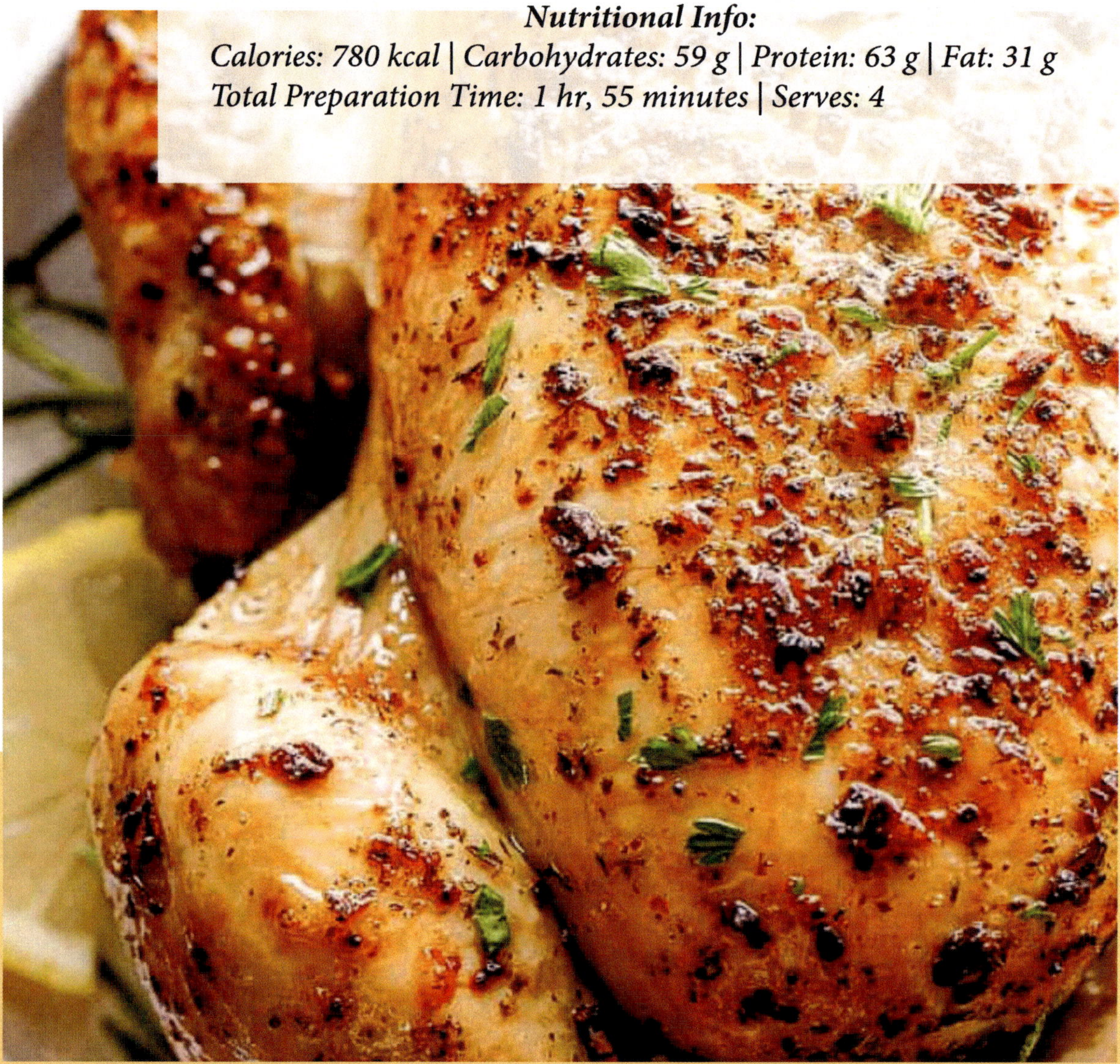

# INGREDIENTS

- *½ cup of onion, chopped*
- *½ cup of celery, chopped*
- *Pinch of ground pepper, to taste*
- *1 tbsp. of butter softened*
- *1 cup of large dry bread cubes*
- *½ tsp. of kosher salt*
- *1 cup of low-sodium hot chicken broth*
- *1 large egg*
- *3 lb. of chicken breast, halved and skin on*
- *3 tsp. of melted fresh butter (for brushing)*
- *Cayenne pepper (to taste)*
- *1 tsp. of poultry seasoning*

# DIRECTIONS

1. In a pan over medium heat, melt 2 tablespoons of butter.
2. Add the onions and celery.
3. Cook for about 6 minutes, or until golden brown.
4. Remove the pan from the heat.
5. Combine the bread cubes, poultry seasoning, sautéed onions, celery, salt, and pepper in a mixing dish.
6. Add the chicken broth and toss until well combined.
7. Allow the mixture to sit for about 15 minutes, to allow the broth to permeate into the stuffing.
8. Stir in the egg yolk, until completely integrated.
9. Preheat the oven to 350°F.
10. Line a rimmed baking sheet with parchment paper.
11. Crosswise slice the chicken breast into ¾ inch slices to the bone (do not cut through the bone).
12. Divide the stuffing mixture evenly between the pieces.
13. Transfer the chicken breast to a prepped baking sheet.
14. Brush the butter over the chicken breast and roast it in a preheated oven for 60 to 75 minutes, or until well-browned.
15. Implant a thermometer with an instant-read probe near the bone. When done, the thermometer should read 150°F (65°C).
16. Remove it from the oven and set aside for 10 minutes.
17. Slice the turkey.
18. Serve and enjoy!

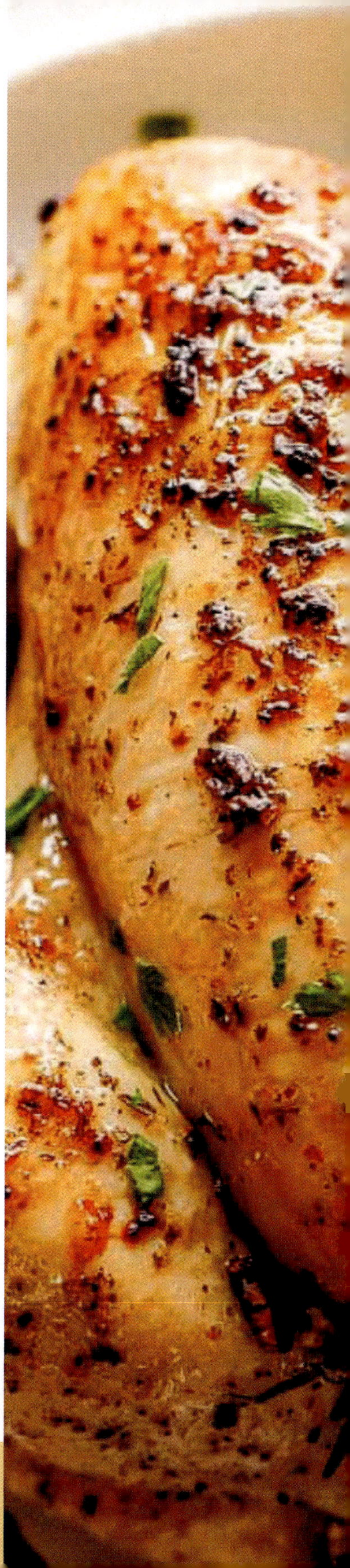

# *Doreen's Ham Slices on the Grill (Grilled Ham Slices)*

**_Nutritional Info:_**

*Calories: 245 kcal | Carbohydrates: 58 g | Protein: 2.7 g | Fat: 1.3 g*

*Total Preparation Time: 25 minutes | Serves: 4*

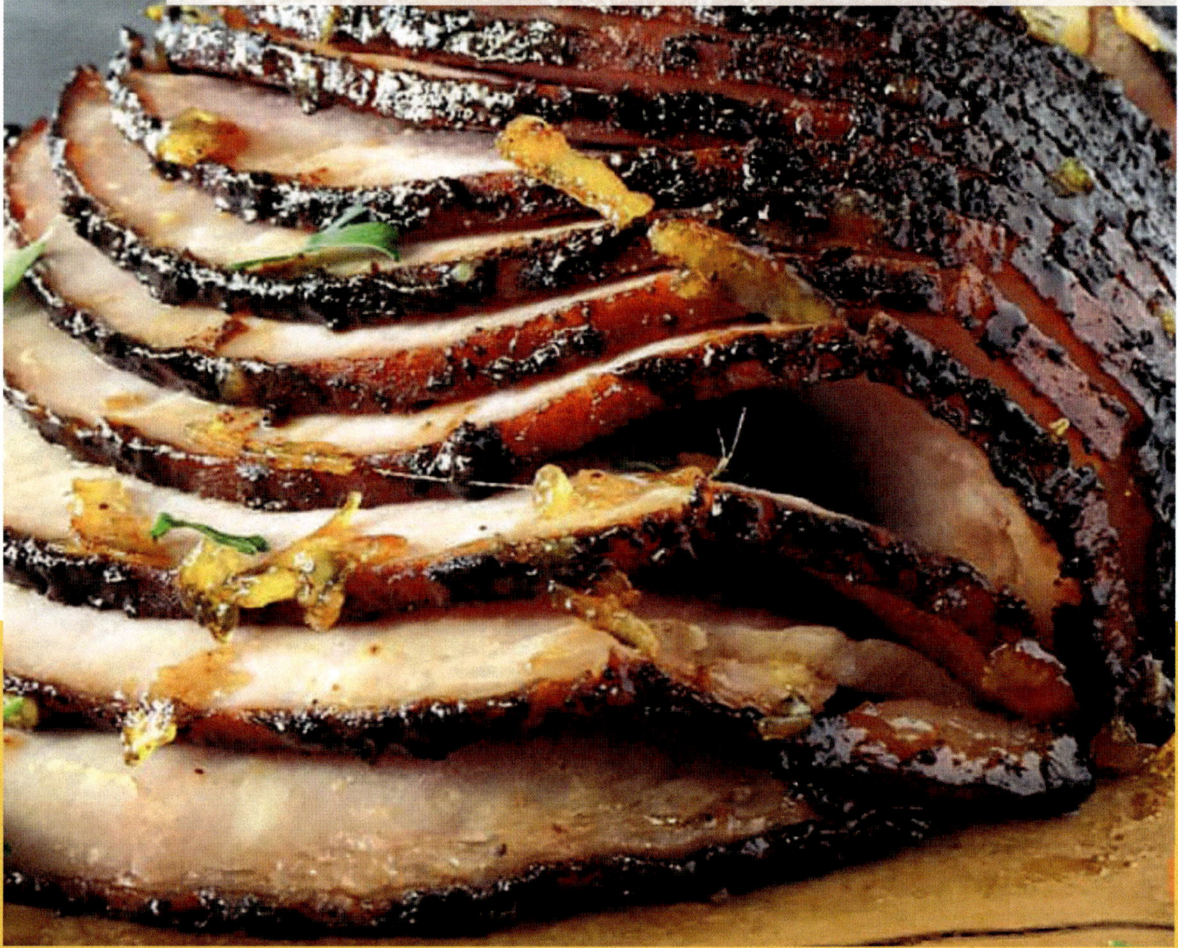

# INGREDIENTS

- *⅓ cup of prepared horseradish*
- *2 ham slices*
- *4 tbsp. of fresh lemon juice*
- *1 cup of packed brown sugar*

# DIRECTIONS

1. Preheat your outside grill to a high temperature and brush the grate gently with oil.
2. Combine the brown sugar, lemon juice, and prepared horseradish in a small bowl.
3. Microwave the brown sugar combination for 1 minute on high, or until heated.
4. Brush the ham slices with the mixture.
5. Arrange the ham slices on the preheated grill.
6. While grilling, regularly baste with the brown sugar mixture.
7. Grill on each side for 7 minutes, or until the desired texture (how done it is) has been achieved.
8. Serve and enjoy!

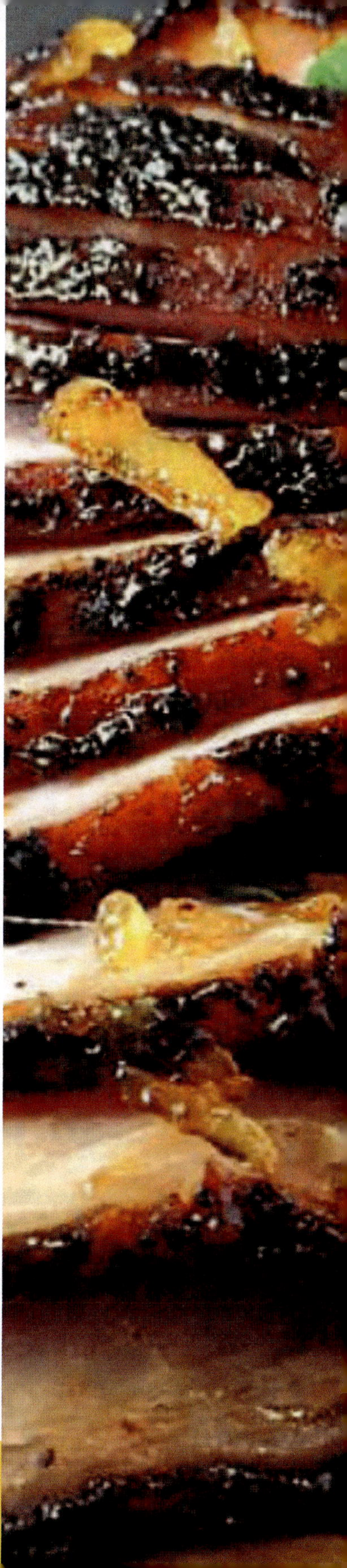

# Pork Steaks with Lemon Butter Sauce

**Nutritional Info:**

*Calories: 173 kcal | Carbohydrates: 0.3 g | Protein: 20.4 g | Fat: 9.5 g*

*Total Preparation Time: 30 minutes | Serves: 6*

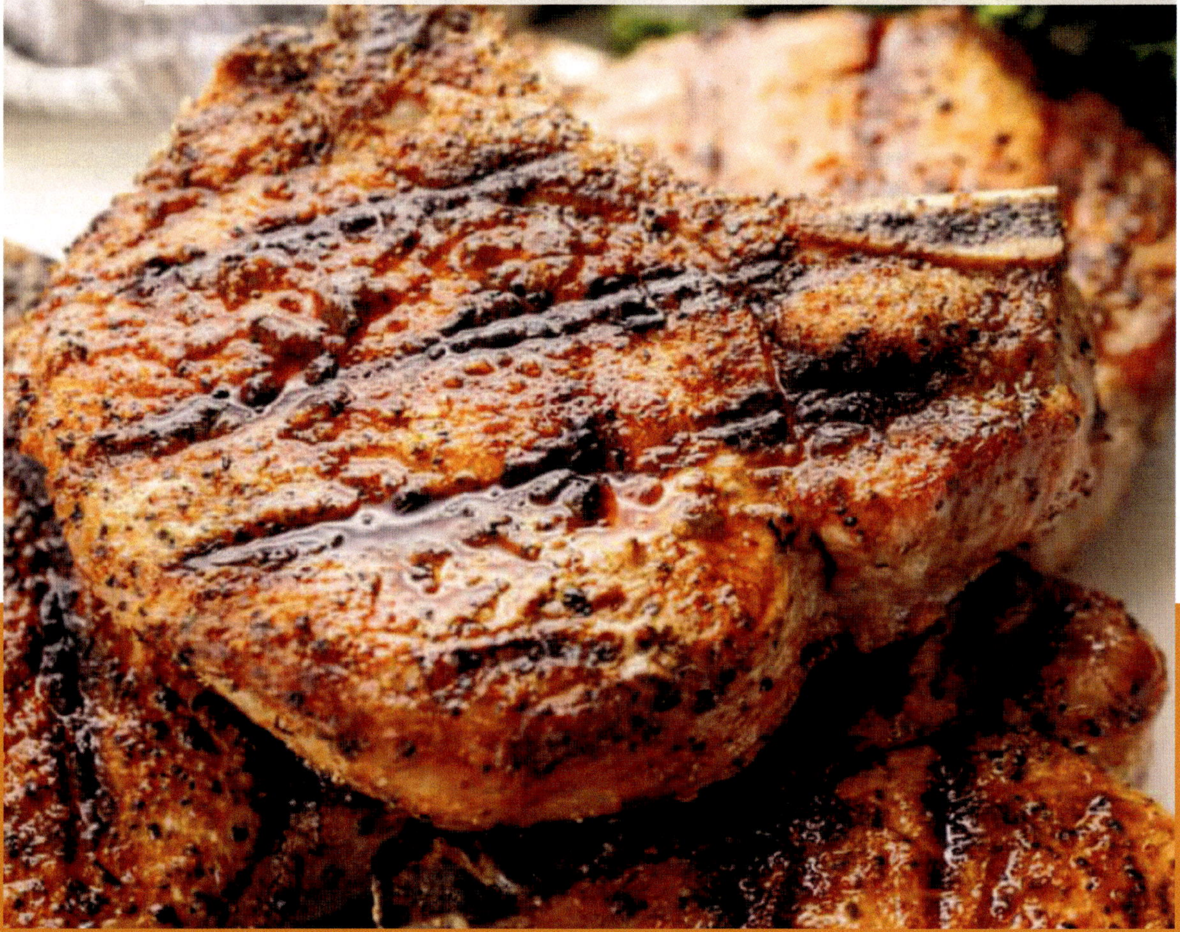

# INGREDIENTS

- *Pinch of kosher salt*
- *3 tbsp. of butter*
- *6 pork chops*
- *2 tsp. of lemon juice*
- *1 clove of garlic, minced*

# DIRECTIONS

1. Preheat your outside grill to a high temperature.
2. Brush the grill gently with oil.
3. Place the small saucepan over medium heat and melt the butter.
4. Add the lemon juice and garlic to the saucepan and and cook, stirring occasionally, until the garlic is soft.
5. Take the pan off the heat.
6. Arrange the chops on a dish and brush the tops of each with the butter mixture.
7. Place the chops on the grill, butter side down.
8. Sear for 1 minute over high heat.
9. Brush| the top side of the chops with the butter mixture as the other side grills. Sear the other side of the chops for 1 minute.
10. Turn the meat over, cover the grill, and cook for an additional 3 to 5 minutes per side, brushing the meat occasionally with the remaining butter mixture.
11. When the internal temperature of the pork chops reaches 145°F, they are done.
12. Serve and enjoy!

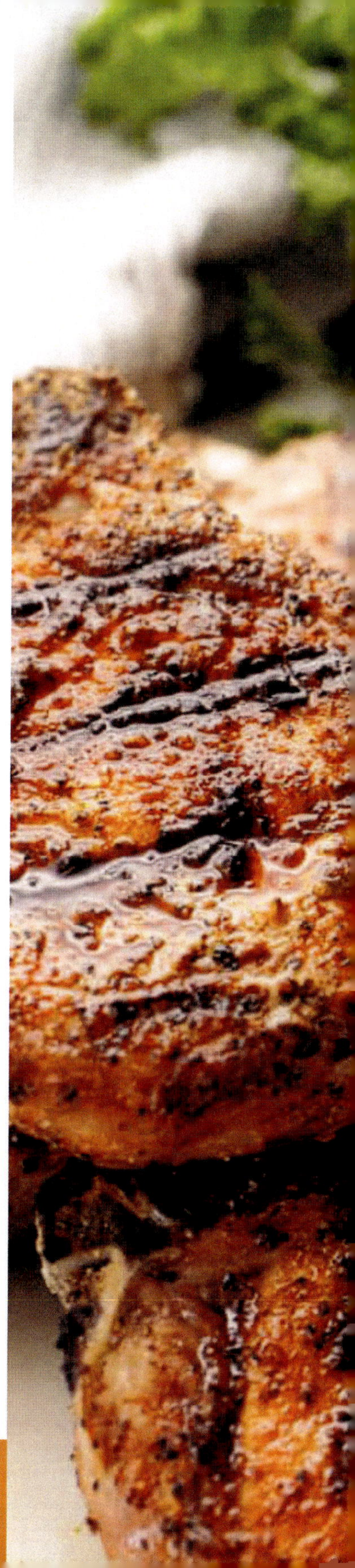

# Christmas Recipes

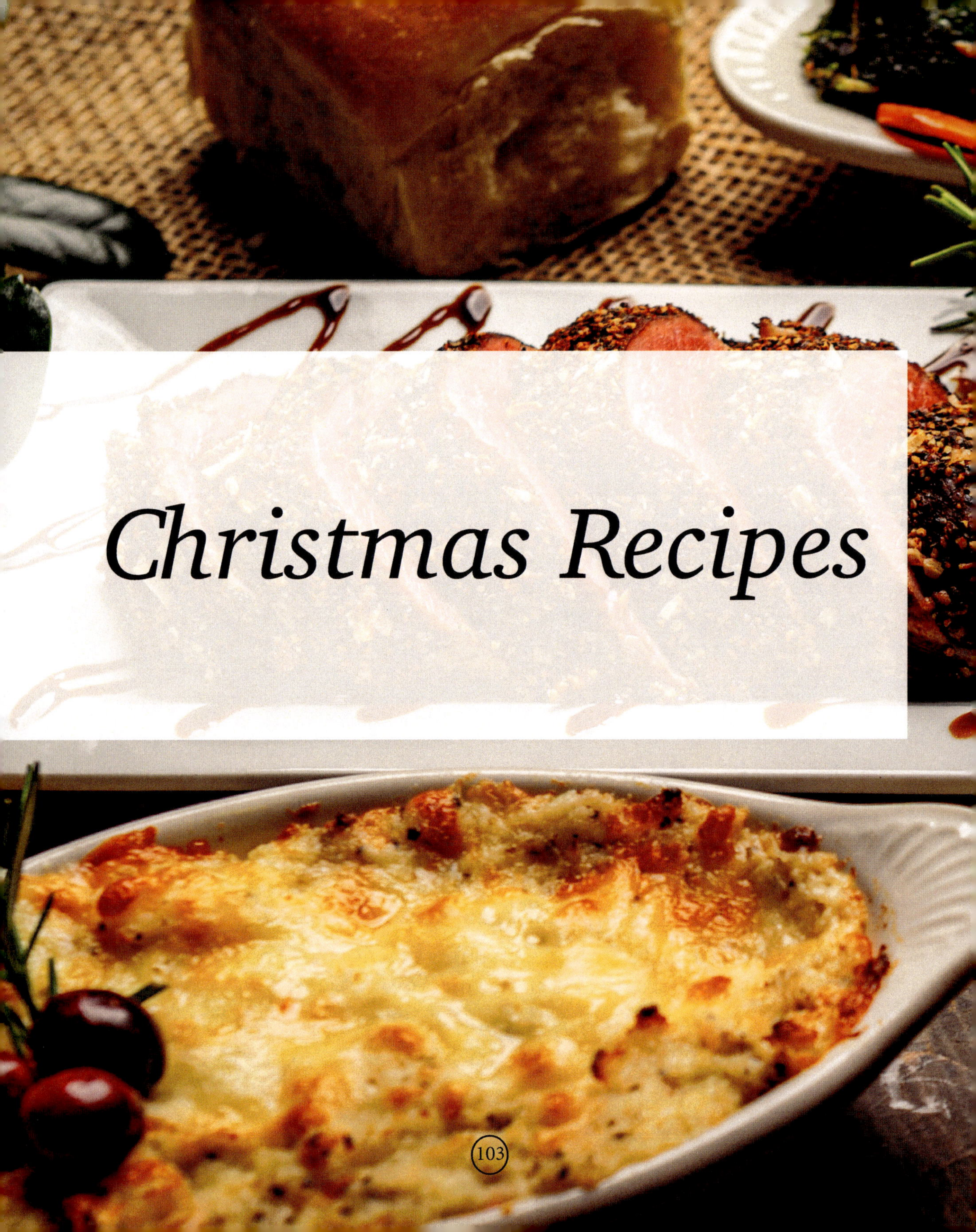

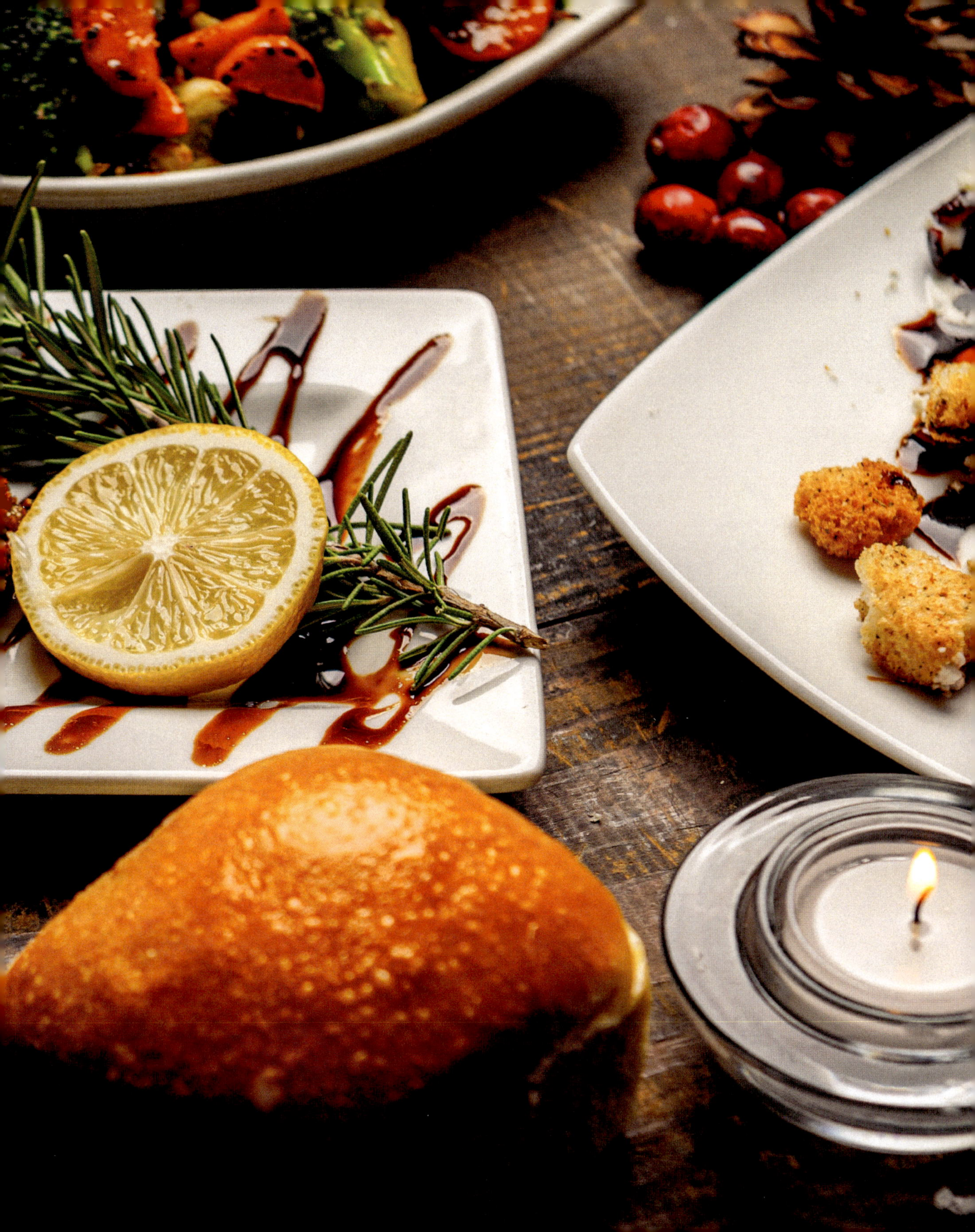

# *Spinach and Ricotta Puff Pastry*

***Nutritional Info:***

*Calories: 246 kcal | Carbohydrates: 19.4 g | Protein: 8 g | Fat: 15.5 g*
*Total Preparation Time: 1 hr, 47 minutes| Serves: 8*

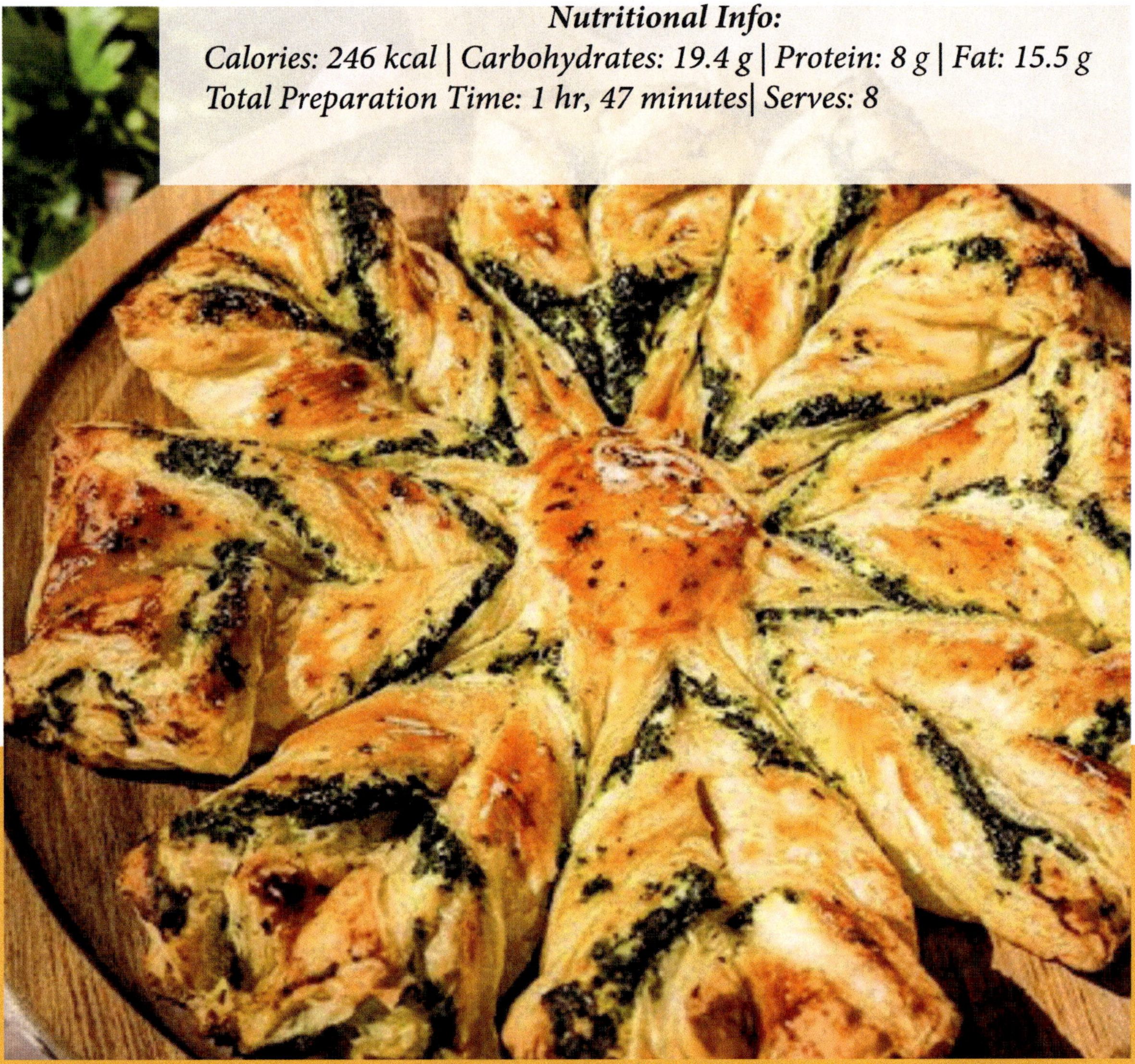

# INGREDIENTS

- *1 tsp. of vegetable oil for cooking*
- *1 sheet of frozen puff pastry, thawed*
- *2 red onions, chopped*
- *9 oz. of fresh ricotta cheese, shredded*
- *1 tbsp. of grated Parmesan cheese, shredded*
- *4 multi-colored cherry tomatoes, halved*
- *8 cups of fresh spinach, chopped*
- *Pinch of ground nutmeg*
- *Salt and freshly ground black pepper*
- *1 egg, lightly beaten*

# DIRECTIONS

1. **Place** the large skillet over medium heat.
2. **Heat** the oil and sauté the onions until tender and transparent.
3. Add spinach, salt, and pepperoni the skillet.
4. **Sauté** for 2 to 3 minutes, stirring regularly.
5. Cover and cook for 5 to 7 minutes, or until spinach has wilted.
6. After 5 minutes, remove the lid and allow the liquid to evaporate.
7. Remove from heat and let it cool completely.
8. In a bowl, combine the spinach mixture and both cheeses.
9. Season the mixture with salt, pepper, and freshly grated nutmeg (according to your taste preference).
10. Roll out the puff pastry sheet and fill it within ½ inch of the edges with the spinach-cheese mixture.
11. Roll the sheet tightly, lengthwise, and firmly press the edges together.
12. Fold in a plastic bag and chill for at least 1 hour in the refrigerator.
13. Preheat the oven to 350°F.
14. Line a baking sheet with parchment paper. Slice pastry logs into ¾ inch slices to create 16 to 22 pinwheels; arrange the puff pastry pinwheels to resemble a Christmas tree. The bottom row should have six pinwheels; the second row should have five; so on, and so forth.
15. If you have with 16 pinwheels, start at the lowest row with 5 pinwheels, and then place the final wheel on the bottom to form the stem.
16. Egg wash and bake for 20 to 25 minutes until golden and puffy. *Additional Option: Cherry tomatoes can be used as Christmas tree ornaments.*
17. Serve and enjoy!

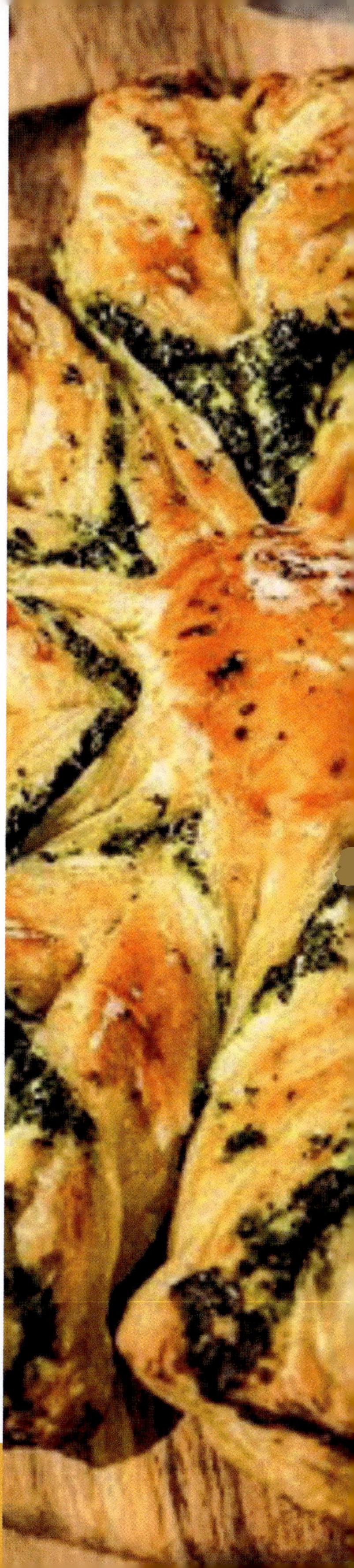

# Broccoli and Bacon Salad with Creamy Dressing

***Nutritional Info:***
*Calories: 250 kcal | Carbohydrates: 28 g | Protein: 3 g | Fat: 14 g*
*Total Preparation Time: 20 minutes | Serves: 8*

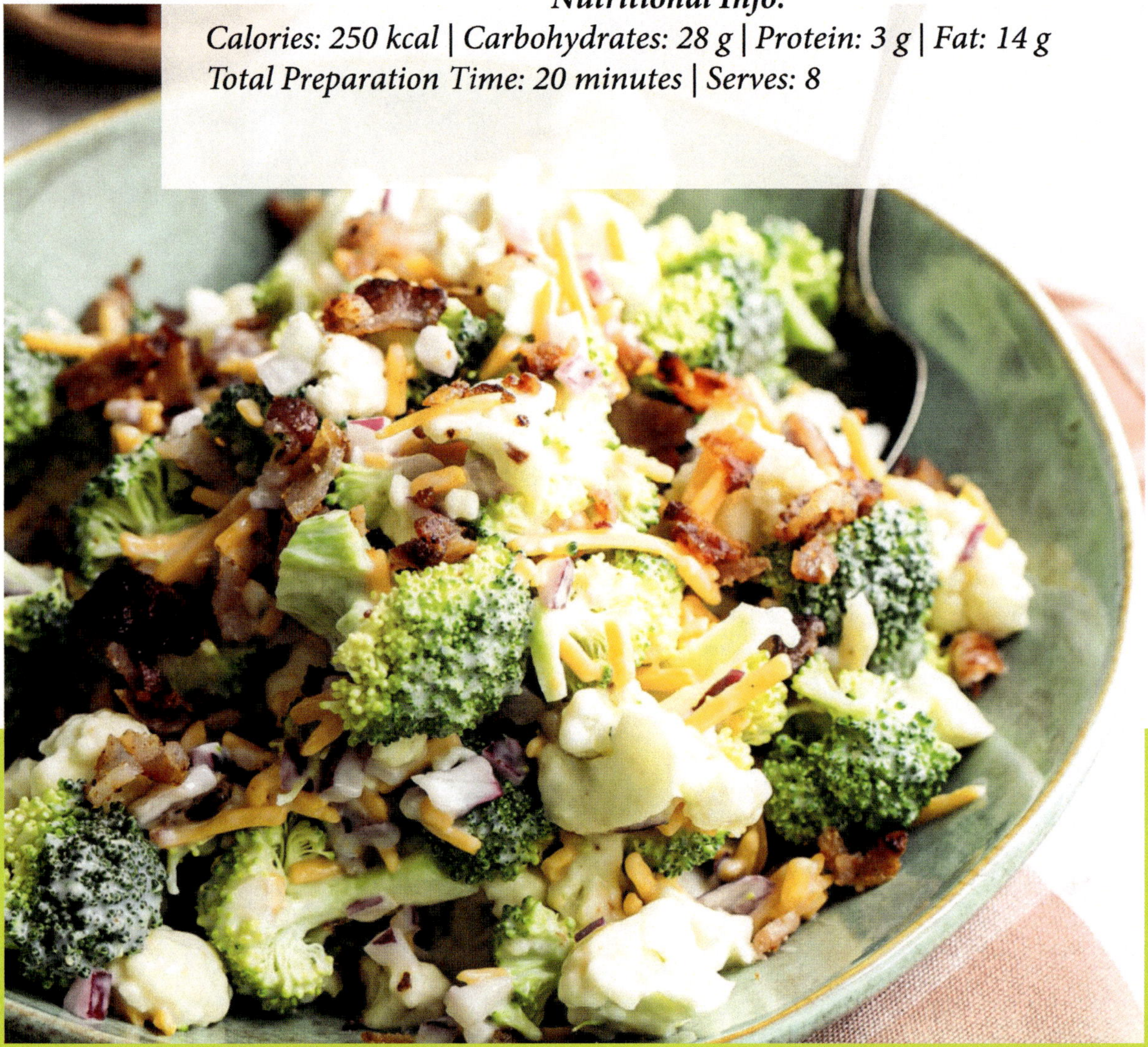

# *INGREDIENTS*

- *150 g of smoked bacon rashers*
- *800 g of broccoli, florets*
- *½ cup of whole-egg mayonnaise*
- *1 tbsp. of lemon juice, freshly squeezed*
- *1 tbsp. of whole grain mustard*
- *1 tsp. of Dijon mustard*
- *¾ cup of red grapes, halved*
- *2 green shallots, thinly sliced*
- *2 tbsp. of toasted slivered almonds*

# *DIRECTIONS*

1. Place the large frying pan over medium-high heat.
2. Add the bacon to the pan and cook for 4-5 minutes, rotating once, or until golden and crisp.
3. Take the bacon out of the pan and chop coarsely.
4. Meanwhile, over high heat, bring a saucepan of water to a boil.
5. Stir in the broccoli and cook for 3-4 minutes, until tender and bright green.
6. Drain the water and then rinse the broccoli in cold water.
7. In a small ceramic bowl, beat together the mayonnaise, lemon juice, and mustard to make the dressing.
8. Arrange the broccoli on a serving tray and season with salt and pepper to taste.
9. Arrange the bacon, grapes, shallot, and nuts on top of the broccoli.
10. Drizzle the dressing over top. (Toss gently to coat, if desired.)
11. Serve and enjoy!

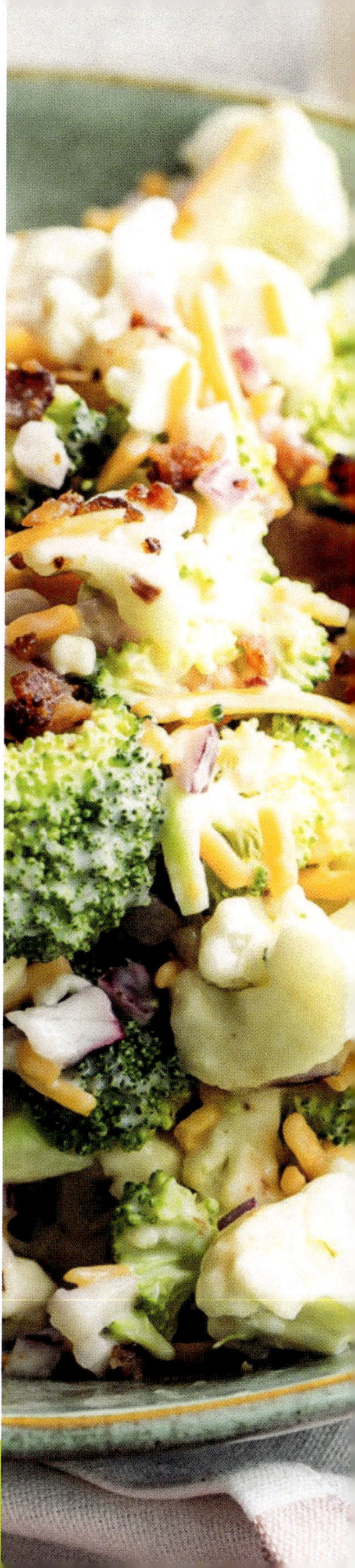

# Basil Ricotta Gnocchi

**Nutritional Info:**

*Calories: 324 kcal | Carbohydrates: 20.2 g | Protein: 19.3 g, Fat: 18.3 g*
*Total Preparation Time: 1 hr, 20 minutes | Serves: 4*

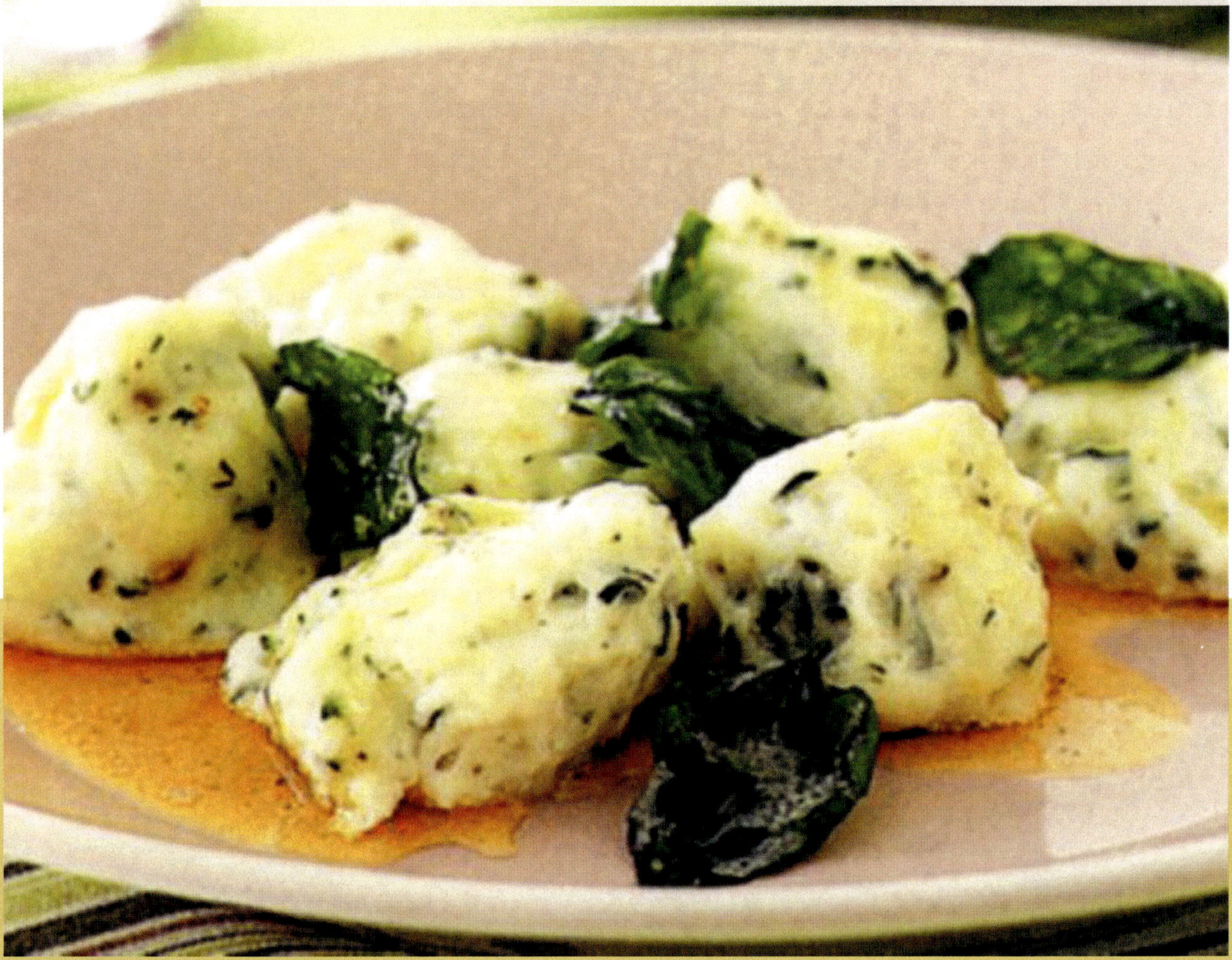

# INGREDIENTS

- *12 oz. of whole milk ricotta cheese*
- *1¼ tsp. of kosher salt*
- *1½ oz. of parmesan cheese, shredded*
- *¾ cup of all-purpose flour*
- *Pinch of cayenne pepper*
- *2 tbsp. of unsalted butter for greasing*
- *2 medium-sized eggs, lightly beaten*
- *1 cup of fresh basil leaves, chopped*

# DIRECTIONS

1. Briefly blanch the basil in simmering water for about 20 seconds.
2. Immediately transfer the basil leaves to a dish of cold water to halt the cooking process.
3. Dry the basil leaves on paper towels.
4. Blend the basil leaves and eggs in a mixing bowl until the basil is completely incorporated and the mixture becomes an even green color with flecks of basil.
5. Add the ricotta cheese to the mixture.
6. Combine the egg mixture, salt, cayenne pepper, parmesan cheese, and flour in a medium bowl.
7. Mix thoroughly with a spatula, ensuring that all ingredients are uniformly distributed.
8. Cover and refrigerate for 2 hours, or until cool and stiff.
9. Scoop a tiny quantity of dough with a teaspoon and shape it into a spherical oval using a second spoon. Repeat until you have about 6 gnocchi for a batch.
10. Bring a big saucepan of salted water to low heat and then bring to a simmer.
11. As you create the gnocchi, drop them into the pot in batches of 6. They will float to the surface after about a minute. It will continue to simmer for 2 to 3 minutes longer.
12. Using a slotted spoon, transfer to a plate to cool. Repeat with the remainder of the dough.

*Additional Option: In a skillet, melt butter until it begins to bubble. Brown each side of the prepared gnocchi. Garnish with shredded parmesan cheese and a drizzle of the pan butter.*

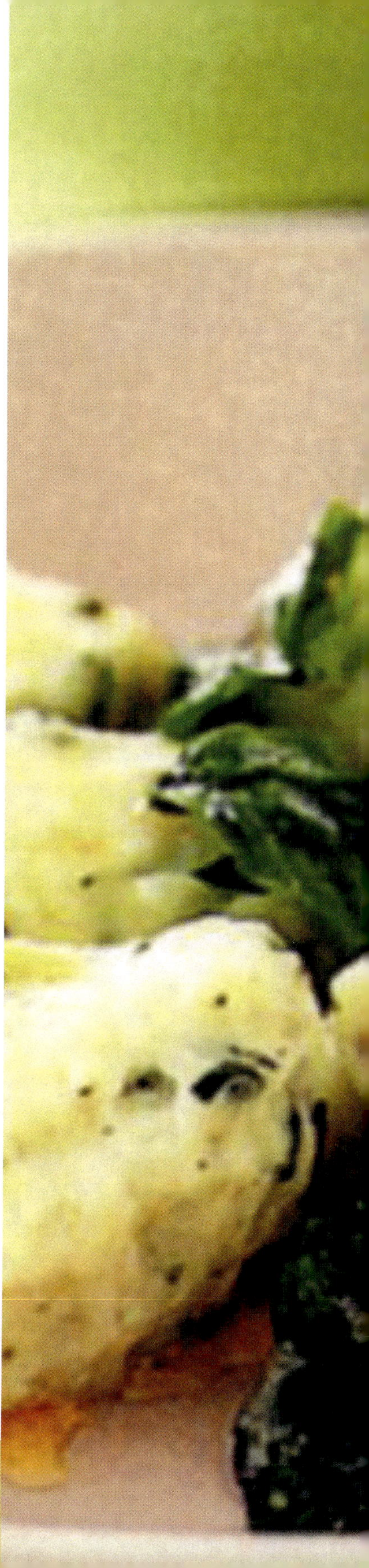

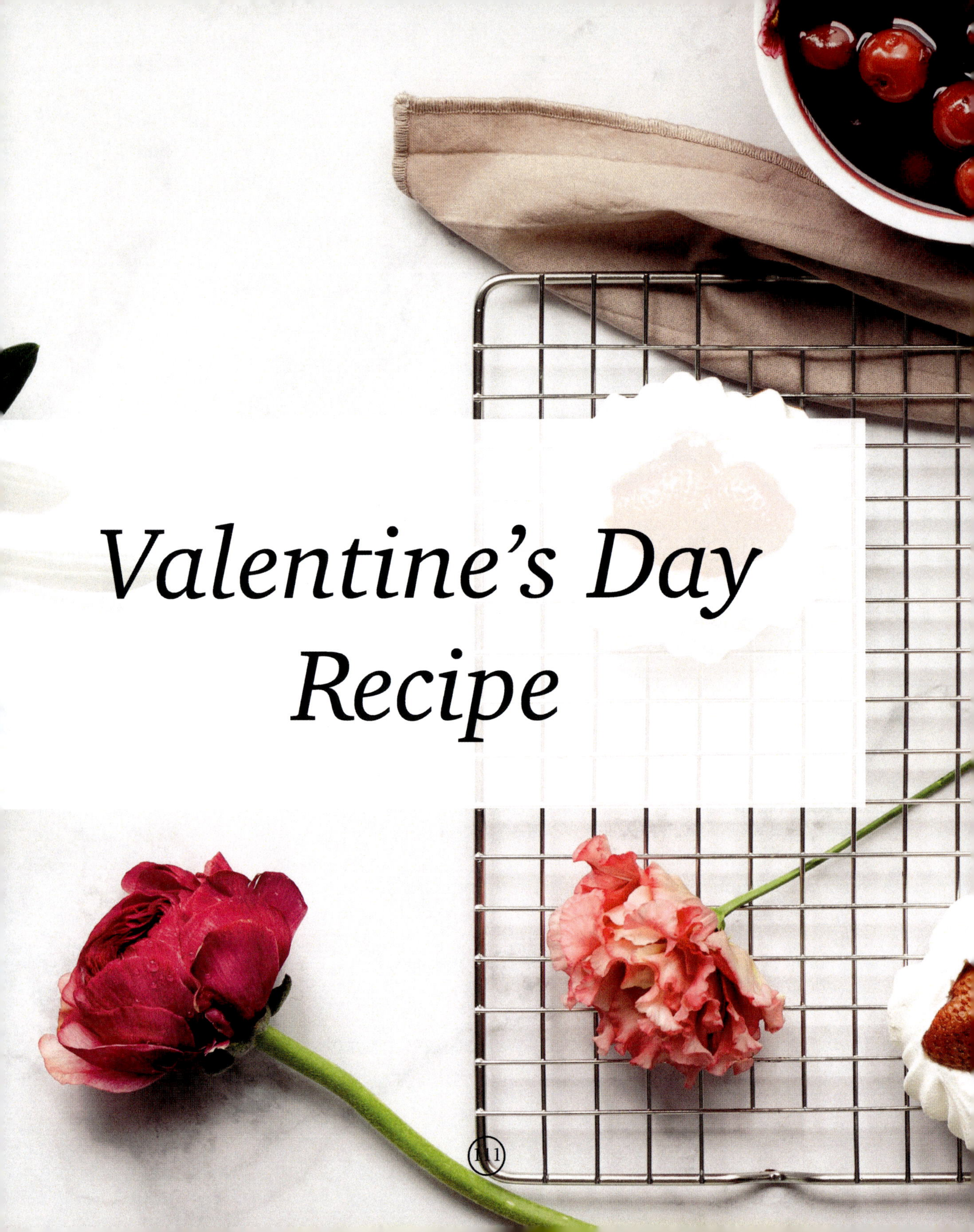

# *Valentine's Day Recipe*

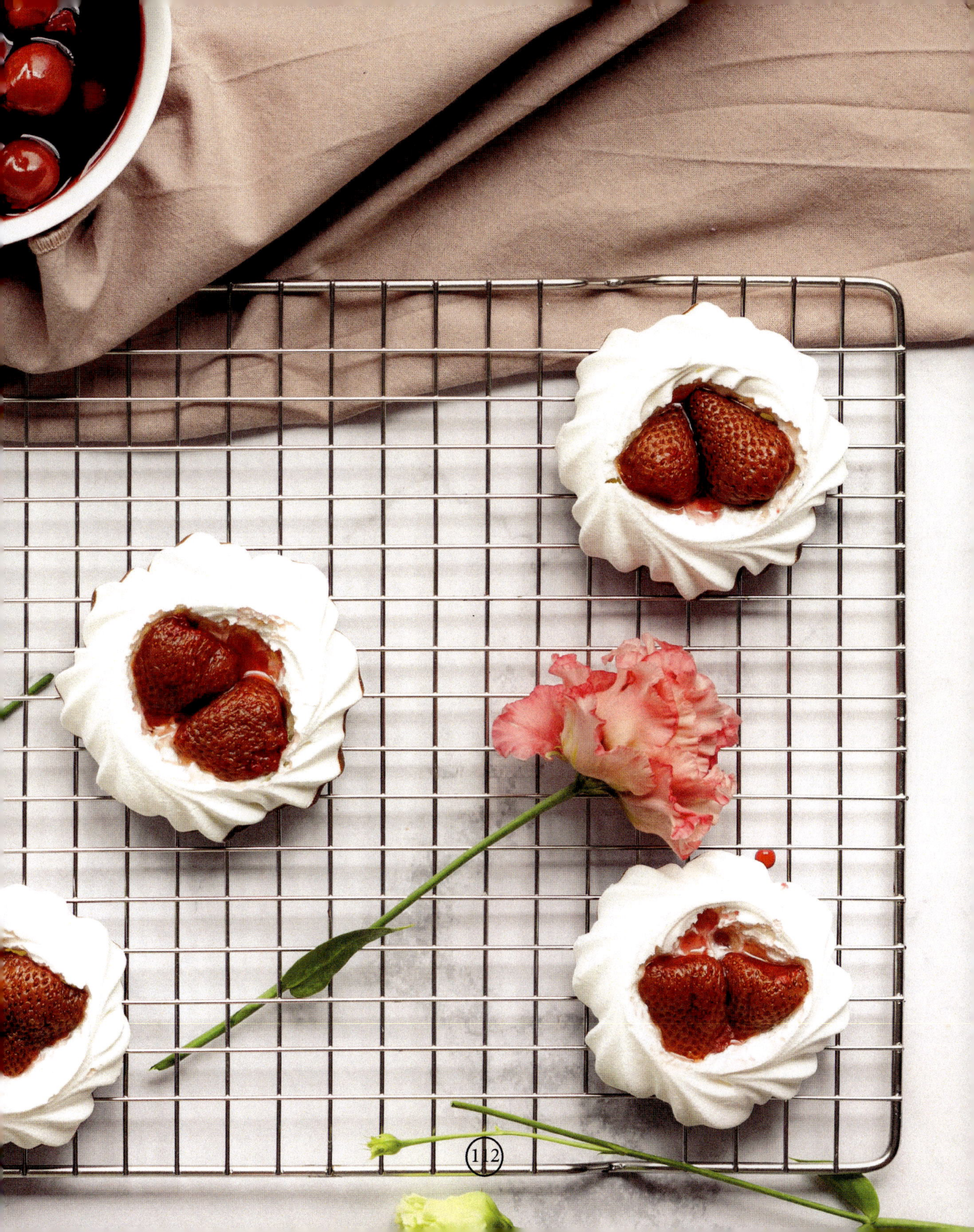

# Strawberries Dipped in Dark Chocolate

LOVE'S HOLISTIC NUTRITION

**Nutritional Info:**

*Calories: 127 kcal | Carbohydrates: 14 g | Fat: 7 g | Protein: 2g*
*Total Preparation Time: 30 minutes | Serves: 4*

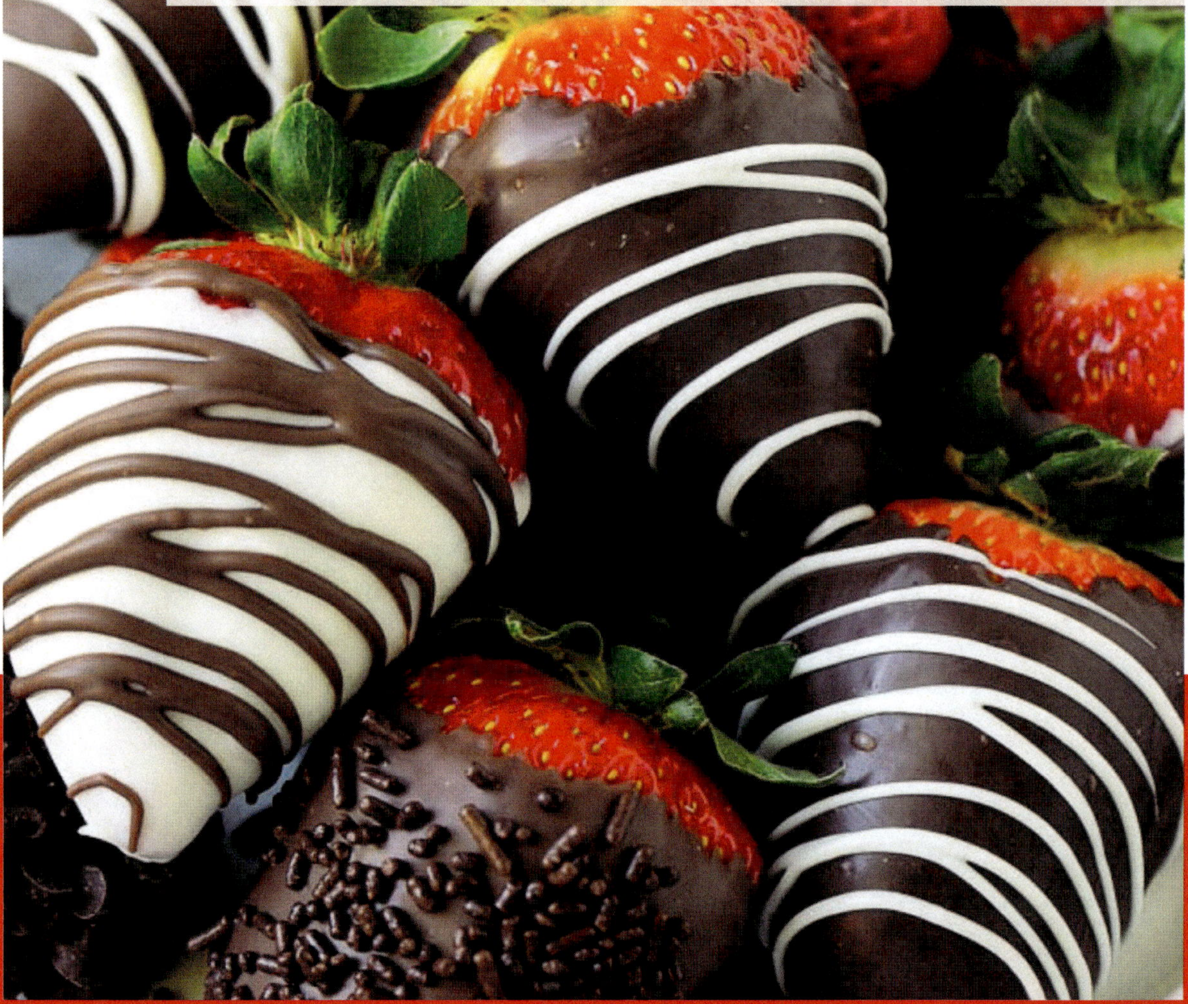

# INGREDIENTS

- *½ cup of strawberries, washed*
- *½ cup of dark chocolate*

# DIRECTIONS

1. Fill the bottom of the double boiler with water.
2. Heat the double boiler (on a high temperature) until it comes to a boil.
3. Turn the heat down to a low temperature.
4. Add the chocolate to the top of the double boiler.
5. Melt the chocolate gradually over the low heat.
6. Once the chocolate is almost smooth, remove it from the burner.
7. Continue stirring the chocolate until it becomes smooth.
8. Slowly roll the strawberry in the chocolate.
9. Hold the strawberry by the top to coat evenly, while leaving a small portion of the fruit visible at the top.
10. For a few moments, invert the strawberry, by allowing the extra chocolate to fall off.
11. Place the chocolate-covered strawberry on wax paper to harden.
12. Refrigerate until ready to eat (at least 30 minutes).
13. Serve and enjoy!

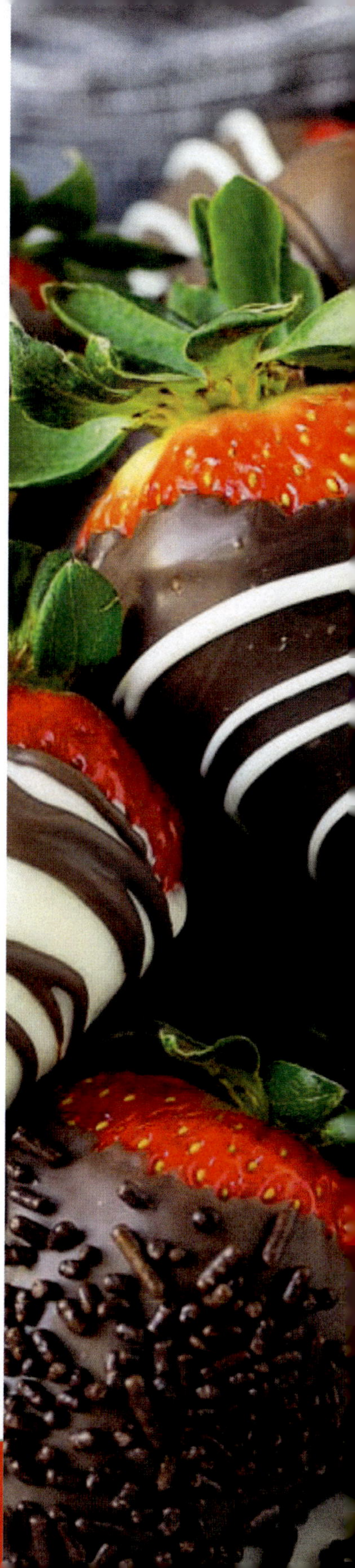

# Daily Food Journal

LOVE'S HOLISTIC NUTRITION

**Wake up time** ______________ **am/pm**

| Time/Meal | Food/ Beverage | Cal. | Pro. | Carb. | Fat. |
|---|---|---|---|---|---|
| | | | | | |
| | | | | | |
| | | | | | |
| | | | | | |
| | | | | | |
| | | | | | |
| | | | | | |
| | | | | | |
| | | | | | |
| | | | | | |
| | | | | | |
| | | | | | |
| | | | | | |
| | | | | | |
| | | | | | |
| | | | | | |
| | **Daily Total** | | | | |
| | **Daily Goal** | | | | |

## Sleep the night before

Bed time: ______________am/pm

# of Hours (      )

How did you sleep ?

## Supplements:

- [ ] Fish oil
- [ ] Polyphenols
- [ ] ..........
- [ ] ..........

## Water: 8 glasses/day

- [ ] 8Oz
- [ ] 8Oz
- [ ] 8Oz
- [ ] 8Oz
- [ ] 8Oz
- [ ] 8Oz
- [ ] 8Oz
- [ ] 8Oz

## Exercise/ Activity

- [ ] Cardio ..........
Time (      )
- [ ] Strength ..........
Time (      )
- [ ] Intervals ..........
Time (      )
- [ ] Other ..........
Time (      )
- [ ] Daily steps ..........

**How do I feel?** (mood, energy level, ability to think clearly, alertness etc.)

# Recipe

Love's Holistic Nutrition

**Name**

**Serves:** ____________

**Prep Time:** ____________

**Rating:** ☆ ☆ ☆ ☆ ☆

**Cook Time:** ____________

## INGREDIENTS

- [ ]
- [ ]
- [ ]
- [ ]
- [ ]
- [ ]
- [ ]
- [ ]
- [ ]
- [ ]
- [ ]
- [ ]
- [ ]
- [ ]
- [ ]
- [ ]

## INSTRUCTIONS

# Daily Food Journal

LOVE'S HOLISTIC NUTRITION

Wake up time ______________ am/pm

| Time/Meal | Food/ Beverage | Cal. | Pro. | Carb. | Fat. |
|---|---|---|---|---|---|
| | | | | | |
| | | | | | |
| | | | | | |
| | | | | | |
| | | | | | |
| | | | | | |
| | | | | | |
| | | | | | |
| | | | | | |
| | | | | | |
| | | | | | |
| | | | | | |
| | | | | | |
| | | | | | |
| | | | | | |
| | | | | | |
| | | | | | |
| | **Daily Total** | | | | |
| | **Daily Goal** | | | | |

## Sleep the night before

Bed time:
______________am/pm

# of Hours (      )

How did you sleep ?

.................................

.................................

.................................

## Supplements:

- ☐ Fish oil
- ☐ Polyphenols
- ☐ .................................
- ☐ .................................

## Water:

8 glasses/day

- ☐ 8Oz ☐ 8Oz
- ☐ 8Oz ☐ 8Oz
- ☐ 8Oz ☐ 8Oz
- ☐ 8Oz ☐ 8Oz

## Exercise/ Activity

- ☐ Cardio .................
  Time (      )
- ☐ Strength .................
  Time (      )
- ☐ Intervals .................
  Time (      )
- ☐ Other .................
  Time (      )
- ☐ Daily steps .................

**How do I feel?** (mood, energy level, ability to think clearly, alertness etc.)

.................................................................................................

.................................................................................................

# Recipe

LOVE'S HOLISTIC NUTRITION

**Name**

**Serves:**

**Prep Time:**

**Rating:** ☆☆☆☆☆

**Cook Time:**

## INGREDIENTS

## INSTRUCTIONS

# Daily Food Journal

LOVE'S HOLISTIC NUTRITION

**Wake up time** ______________ **am/pm**

| Time/Meal | Food/ Beverage | Cal. | Pro. | Carb. | Fat. |
|---|---|---|---|---|---|
| | | | | | |
| | | | | | |
| | | | | | |
| | | | | | |
| | | | | | |
| | | | | | |
| | | | | | |
| | | | | | |
| | | | | | |
| | | | | | |
| | | | | | |
| | | | | | |
| | | | | | |
| | | | | | |
| | | | | | |
| | | | | | |
| | | | | | |
| | **Daily Total** | | | | |
| | **Daily Goal** | | | | |

## Sleep the night before

Bed time:
______________am/pm

# of Hours (      )

How did you sleep ?

## Supplements:

- ☐ Fish oil
- ☐ Polyphenols
- ☐
- ☐

## Water:

8 glasses/day

| | |
|---|---|
| ☐ 8Oz | ☐ 8Oz |
| ☐ 8Oz | ☐ 8Oz |
| ☐ 8Oz | ☐ 8Oz |
| ☐ 8Oz | ☐ 8Oz |

## Exercise/ Activity

☐ Cardio
Time (      )

☐ Strength
Time (      )

☐ Intervals
Time (      )

☐ Other
Time (      )

☐ Daily steps

**How do I feel?** (mood, energy level, ability to think clearly, alertness etc.)

# Recipe

Love's Holistic Nutrition

**Name**

**Serves:** ____________________ **Prep Time:** ____________________

**Rating:** ☆☆☆☆☆ **Cook Time:** ____________________

## INGREDIENTS

- ○
- ○
- ○
- ○
- ○
- ○
- ○
- ○
- ○
- ○
- ○
- ○
- ○
- ○
- ○
- ○

## INSTRUCTIONS

# Daily Food Journal

Love's Holistic Nutrition

**Wake up time ______________ am/pm**

| Time/Meal | Food/ Beverage | Cal. | Pro. | Carb. | Fat. |
|---|---|---|---|---|---|
| | | | | | |
| | | | | | |
| | | | | | |
| | | | | | |
| | | | | | |
| | | | | | |
| | | | | | |
| | | | | | |
| | | | | | |
| | | | | | |
| | | | | | |
| | | | | | |
| | | | | | |
| | | | | | |
| | | | | | |
| | | | | | |
| | | | | | |
| | | | | | |
| | **Daily Total** | | | | |
| | **Daily Goal** | | | | |

## Sleep the night before

Bed time:

____________am/pm

\# of Hours (    )

How did you sleep ?

## Supplements:

- ☐ Fish oil
- ☐ Polyphenols
- ☐
- ☐

## Water:

8 glasses/day

| | |
|---|---|
| ☐ 8Oz | ☐ 8Oz |
| ☐ 8Oz | ☐ 8Oz |
| ☐ 8Oz | ☐ 8Oz |
| ☐ 8Oz | ☐ 8Oz |

## Exercise/ Activity

☐ Cardio

Time (    )

☐ Strength

Time (    )

☐ Intervals

Time (    )

☐ Other

Time (    )

☐ Daily steps

**How do I feel?** (mood, energy level, ability to think clearly, alertness etc.)

# Recipe

LOVE'S HOLISTIC NUTRITION

**Name**

**Serves:**

**Prep Time:**

**Rating:** ☆☆☆☆☆

**Cook Time:**

## INGREDIENTS

## INSTRUCTIONS

# Daily Food Journal

Love's Holistic Nutrition

**Wake up time** ______________ **am/pm**

| Time/Meal | Food/ Beverage | Cal. | Pro. | Carb. | Fat. |
|---|---|---|---|---|---|
| | | | | | |
| | | | | | |
| | | | | | |
| | | | | | |
| | | | | | |
| | | | | | |
| | | | | | |
| | | | | | |
| | | | | | |
| | | | | | |
| | | | | | |
| | | | | | |
| | | | | | |
| | | | | | |
| | | | | | |
| | | | | | |
| | | | | | |
| | **Daily Total** | | | | |
| | **Daily Goal** | | | | |

## Sleep the night before

**Bed time:**
____________am/pm

**# of Hours (      )**

**How did you sleep ?**

................................

................................

................................

## Supplements:

- ☐ Fish oil
- ☐ Polyphenols
- ☐ ................
- ☐ ................

## Water:

8 glasses/day

- ☐ 8Oz ☐ 8Oz
- ☐ 8Oz ☐ 8Oz
- ☐ 8Oz ☐ 8Oz
- ☐ 8Oz ☐ 8Oz

## Exercise/ Activity

- ☐ Cardio ................
  Time (      )
- ☐ Strength ................
  Time (      )
- ☐ Intervals ................
  Time (      )
- ☐ Other ................
  Time (      )
- ☐ Daily steps ................

**How do I feel?** (mood, energy level, ability to think clearly, alertness etc.)

................................................................................

................................................................................

# Recipe

LOVE'S HOLISTIC NUTRITION

**Name**

**Serves:** ________________ **Prep Time:** ________________

**Rating:** ☆☆☆☆☆ **Cook Time:** ________________

## INGREDIENTS

○ ○
○ ○
○ ○
○ ○
○ ○
○ ○
○ ○
○ ○

## INSTRUCTIONS

# Daily Food Journal

LOVE'S HOLISTIC NUTRITION

**Wake up time** ______________ **am/pm**

| Time/Meal | Food/ Beverage | Cal. | Pro. | Carb. | Fat. |
|---|---|---|---|---|---|
| | | | | | |
| | | | | | |
| | | | | | |
| | | | | | |
| | | | | | |
| | | | | | |
| | | | | | |
| | | | | | |
| | | | | | |
| | | | | | |
| | | | | | |
| | | | | | |
| | | | | | |
| | | | | | |
| | | | | | |
| | | | | | |
| | | | | | |
| | **Daily Total** | | | | |
| | **Daily Goal** | | | | |

## Sleep the night before

Bed time:
____________am/pm

# of Hours (      )

How did you sleep ?

## Supplements:

- ☐ Fish oil
- ☐ Polyphenols
- ☐
- ☐

## Water:

8 glasses/day

- ☐ 8Oz ☐ 8Oz
- ☐ 8Oz ☐ 8Oz
- ☐ 8Oz ☐ 8Oz
- ☐ 8Oz ☐ 8Oz

## Exercise/ Activity

- ☐ Cardio
  Time (      )
- ☐ Strength
  Time (      )
- ☐ Intervals
  Time (      )
- ☐ Other
  Time (      )
- ☐ Daily steps

**How do I feel?** (mood, energy level, ability to think clearly, alertness etc.)

# Recipe

Love's Holistic Nutrition

**Name**

**Serves:** ______________________

**Prep Time:** ______________________

**Rating:** ☆ ☆ ☆ ☆ ☆

**Cook Time:** ______________________

## INGREDIENTS

○ ○
○ ○
○ ○
○ ○
○ ○
○ ○
○ ○
○ ○

## INSTRUCTIONS

# Daily Food Journal

Love's Holistic Nutrition

**Wake up time** ______________ **am/pm**

| Time/Meal | Food/ Beverage | Cal. | Pro. | Carb. | Fat. |
|---|---|---|---|---|---|
| | | | | | |
| | | | | | |
| | | | | | |
| | | | | | |
| | | | | | |
| | | | | | |
| | | | | | |
| | | | | | |
| | | | | | |
| | | | | | |
| | | | | | |
| | | | | | |
| | | | | | |
| | | | | | |
| | | | | | |
| | | | | | |
| | | | | | |
| | **Daily Total** | | | | |
| | **Daily Goal** | | | | |

## Sleep the night before

Bed time: ______________am/pm

# of Hours (    )

How did you sleep ?

................................................

................................................

................................................

## Supplements:

- ☐ Fish oil
- ☐ Polyphenols
- ☐ ................................
- ☐ ................................

## Water:

8 glasses/day

☐ 8Oz ☐ 8Oz

☐ 8Oz ☐ 8Oz

☐ 8Oz ☐ 8Oz

☐ 8Oz ☐ 8Oz

## Exercise/ Activity

☐ Cardio ....................

Time (    )

☐ Strength ....................

Time (    )

☐ Intervals ....................

Time (    )

☐ Other ....................

Time (    )

☐ Daily steps ....................

**How do I feel?** (mood, energy level, ability to think clearly, alertness etc.)

................................................................................................

................................................................................................

# Recipe

LOVE'S HOLISTIC NUTRITION

**Name**

**Serves:** ______________________

**Prep Time:** ______________________

**Rating:** ☆ ☆ ☆ ☆ ☆

**Cook Time:** ______________________

## INGREDIENTS

- ○
- ○
- ○
- ○
- ○
- ○
- ○
- ○
- ○
- ○
- ○
- ○
- ○
- ○
- ○
- ○

## INSTRUCTIONS

# Daily Food Journal

Love's Holistic Nutrition

Wake up time ______________ am/pm

| Time/Meal | Food/ Beverage | Cal. | Pro. | Carb. | Fat. |
|---|---|---|---|---|---|
| | | | | | |
| | | | | | |
| | | | | | |
| | | | | | |
| | | | | | |
| | | | | | |
| | | | | | |
| | | | | | |
| | | | | | |
| | | | | | |
| | | | | | |
| | | | | | |
| | | | | | |
| | | | | | |
| | | | | | |
| | | | | | |
| | | | | | |
| | Daily Total | | | | |
| | Daily Goal | | | | |

## Sleep the night before

Bed time:
______________am/pm

# of Hours (      )

How did you sleep ?

.................................

.................................

.................................

## Supplements:

- ☐ Fish oil
- ☐ Polyphenols
- ☐ ..........
- ☐ ..........

## Water:

8 glasses/day

- ☐ 8Oz ☐ 8Oz
- ☐ 8Oz ☐ 8Oz
- ☐ 8Oz ☐ 8Oz
- ☐ 8Oz ☐ 8Oz

## Exercise/ Activity

- ☐ Cardio ..........
  Time (      )
- ☐ Strength ..........
  Time (      )
- ☐ Intervals ..........
  Time (      )
- ☐ Other ..........
  Time (      )
- ☐ Daily steps ..........

**How do I feel?** (mood, energy level, ability to think clearly, alertness etc.)

.................................

.................................

# Recipe

Love's Holistic Nutrition

**Name**

**Serves:** ______ **Prep Time:** ______

**Rating:** ☆ ☆ ☆ ☆ ☆ **Cook Time:** ______

## INGREDIENTS

- ○
- ○
- ○
- ○
- ○
- ○
- ○
- ○
- ○
- ○
- ○
- ○
- ○
- ○
- ○
- ○

## INSTRUCTIONS

# Daily Food Journal

LOVE'S HOLISTIC NUTRITION

**Wake up time** ______________ **am/pm**

| Time/Meal | Food/ Beverage | Cal. | Pro. | Carb. | Fat. |
|---|---|---|---|---|---|
| | | | | | |
| | | | | | |
| | | | | | |
| | | | | | |
| | | | | | |
| | | | | | |
| | | | | | |
| | | | | | |
| | | | | | |
| | | | | | |
| | | | | | |
| | | | | | |
| | | | | | |
| | | | | | |
| | | | | | |
| | | | | | |
| | | | | | |
| | **Daily Total** | | | | |
| | **Daily Goal** | | | | |

## Sleep the night before

**Bed time:**
______________ **am/pm**

**# of Hours (   )**

**How did you sleep ?**

## Supplements:

- [ ] Fish oil
- [ ] Polyphenols
- [ ] ..........
- [ ] ..........

## Water:

**8 glasses/day**

- [ ] 8Oz
- [ ] 8Oz
- [ ] 8Oz
- [ ] 8Oz
- [ ] 8Oz
- [ ] 8Oz
- [ ] 8Oz
- [ ] 8Oz

## Exercise/ Activity

- [ ] Cardio ..........
Time (   )
- [ ] Strength ..........
Time (   )
- [ ] Intervals ..........
Time (   )
- [ ] Other ..........
Time (   )

- [ ] Daily steps ..........

**How do I feel?** (mood, energy level, ability to think clearly, alertness etc.)

# Recipe

LOVE'S HOLISTIC NUTRITION

**Name**

**Serves:** ______________________ **Prep Time:** ______________________

**Rating:** ☆ ☆ ☆ ☆ ☆ **Cook Time:** ______________________

## INGREDIENTS

- ○
- ○
- ○
- ○
- ○
- ○
- ○
- ○
- ○
- ○
- ○
- ○
- ○
- ○
- ○
- ○

## INSTRUCTIONS

# Daily Food Journal

LOVE'S HOLISTIC NUTRITION

**Wake up time** ______________ **am/pm**

| Time/Meal | Food/ Beverage | Cal. | Pro. | Carb. | Fat. |
|---|---|---|---|---|---|
| | | | | | |
| | | | | | |
| | | | | | |
| | | | | | |
| | | | | | |
| | | | | | |
| | | | | | |
| | | | | | |
| | | | | | |
| | | | | | |
| | | | | | |
| | | | | | |
| | | | | | |
| | | | | | |
| | | | | | |
| | | | | | |
| | | | | | |
| | | | | | |
| | **Daily Total** | | | | |
| | **Daily Goal** | | | | |

## Sleep the night before

Bed time:
__________am/pm

# of Hours (    )

How did you sleep ?

..........

..........

..........

## Supplements:

- [ ] Fish oil
- [ ] Polyphenols
- [ ] ..........
- [ ] ..........

## Water:

8 glasses/day

- [ ] 8Oz
- [ ] 8Oz
- [ ] 8Oz
- [ ] 8Oz
- [ ] 8Oz
- [ ] 8Oz
- [ ] 8Oz
- [ ] 8Oz

## Exercise/ Activity

- [ ] Cardio ..........
Time (    )
- [ ] Strength ..........
Time (    )
- [ ] Intervals ..........
Time (    )
- [ ] Other ..........
Time (    )
- [ ] Daily steps ..........

**How do I feel?** (mood, energy level, ability to think clearly, alertness etc.)

..........

..........

# Recipe

Love's Holistic Nutrition

**Name**

**Serves:** __________ **Prep Time:** __________

**Rating:** ☆☆☆☆☆ **Cook Time:** __________

## INGREDIENTS

## INSTRUCTIONS

# STAY IN TOUCH WITH CRYSTAL LOVE

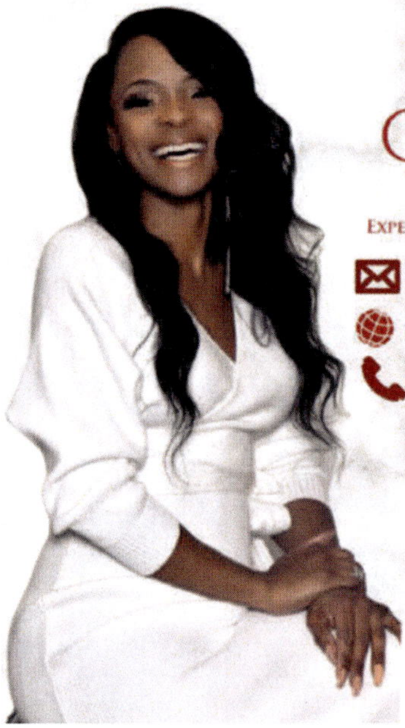

CRYSTAL LOVE
THE AUTHOR

EXPERIENCE LOVE | EMBRACE HEALING | DISCOVER PURPOSE


hello@crystallove-theauthor.com

crystallove-theauthor.com

301-615-4048


SCAN ME

SCAN ME

**Vision Planning**

SCAN ME

**Hair Chemistry**

SCAN ME

SCAN ME

**Meal Plans**

**Counseling**

SCAN ME

LOVE'S HOLISTIC NUTRITION

Made in the USA
Middletown, DE
28 February 2022

61950607R00080